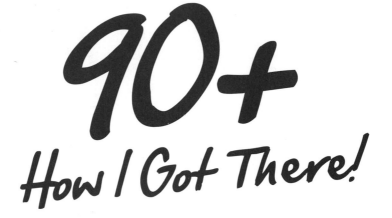

90+
How I Got There!

W. GIFFORD-JONES, MD

ActNatural Corporation
5948 3rd Line RR#1
Hillsburgh, ON
N0B 1Z0

ISBN: 978-0-9867247-8-7

Copy Writing: W. Gifford-Jones, MD
Copy Editing: Karen Gasbarino-Knutt
Cover Photo: Sam Truax
Book and Cover Design: Jasper van Meurs

Printed in Canada by Friesens Corp.

This above all: to thine own self be true,
And it must follow as the night the day,
Thou canst not then be false to any man.

- William Shakespeare

Contents

Foreword
Another book?

I often recall the remark of my ship's captain each and every time we entered a new port. "One more port," he'd sigh. Now I might repeat the expression, substituting "book" for the word port. I have already authored eight books. And when Deane Parkes, President of Preferred Nutrition, urged me to write number 9, I wondered what more I had to say. Weeks later when I was reminded of something I do not like to dwell on, my age of 90+, and how I got there, I thought it might be of interest to others who want to live long and well. The next thought was also disturbing. Since I was already 90+ I shouldn't wait too long to write number 9! Or it would end up like Beethoven's unfinished symphony.

George Bernard Shaw once remarked that "The single biggest problem in communication is the illusion it has taken place." Today the biggest problem with communication in medicine is that it's the wrong communication, often being delivered to medical consumers with disastrous results. During the latter years of my surgical practice, I began to realize that big pharma had created a culture of "consumer pillitis" wherein every minor problem required a pill. But no mention was made of unintended consequences. This triggered my interest in natural remedies that had stood the test of time. They have not killed anyone. Prescription drugs, on the other hand, have removed 100,000 North Americans from this planet every year.

As a medical journalist I've enjoyed the privilege of interviewing international medical authorities. This had a profound influence on my approach to medical matters. And there's no doubt my two lengthy interviews with Dr. Linus Pauling are one of the reasons for writing number 9. I believe Pauling's views on vitamin C, and those of Dr. Sydney Bush, represent to me the greatest medical achievement since I graduated 65 years ago from The Harvard Medical School. It may have the potential to help mankind as much as, or more than, any other research. But is still collecting dust in the medical community. It's an appalling tragedy as their findings of C's benefits could save countless lives.

Voltaire, who spent time in the French prison Bastille once wrote, "It is dangerous to be right, when the government is wrong." During my lifetime as a surgeon and medical journalist I learned that Voltaire was right. When my newspaper column tackled controversial medical topics, my popularity with some segments of society and the medical establishment was jeopardized. The written word is dangerous. But as a journalist one should never expect to win a popularity contest.

Reporting the facts of medicine is never easy. Multinational companies producing chemical therapies are making billions of dollars supposedly to reduce suffering. But they confuse the public, about the cause of heart disease and other medical problems. But sooner or later the truth does emerge. As Winston Churchill wrote, "The truth is inconvertible. Panic may resent it, ignorance may deride it, malice may distort it. But there it is."

In 2015 the truth is that many of us are getting older and living longer. But we all want to live longer well. In this age of degenerative disease the Gifford-Jones Law states that one bad problem leads to another and another. It's best to avoid them as much as possible. Due to faulty lifestyle decisions, obesity may lead to Type 2 diabetes. Its complications may lead to loss of

limbs, blindness and kidney failure. Atherosclerosis due to diabetes may lead to heart attack and sudden death. All may prevent a lengthy and active life.

I hope that this book will show how these disasters and other
medical pitfalls do not have to happen. They will occur less often
if North Americans learn that smart people do at the start of life
what fools attempt at the end.

Enough said.

W. Gifford-Jones, MD

Pitfalls of Lifestyle
Dying Rich at 45

As a boy I spent many hours in Sunday School and church services. So what did I learn? Looking back, I would have preferred to be outside playing. But I have never forgotten one biblical maxim which I was taught. "What will it profit a man if he gains the whole world and loses his own soul?" The tragedy is that of the man who goes through life totally immoral, stealing and cheating to gain great wealth but departs this planet unhappy, unloved and alone. As I look at the medical scene today I see a similar scenario, equally disturbing, that has become a part of our fast-paced materialistic world. As a result, I'd suggest, "What will it profit a man or woman if he or she works diligently to achieve financial success and then dies prematurely of a needless disease?"

It's a story I've seen all too often; Patients who are extremely bright, yet babes in the woods when it comes to medical matters. In fact, some of their pitfalls, stubbornness and irresponsibility are so obvious that it is unbelievable that they happen.

I vividly recall one 45 year old friend and patient who repeatedly refused my advice to have a colonoscopy done. His usual remark was, "They're not going to do that to me!" A few years later he noticed rectal bleeding and still would not agree to this life-saving procedure. Unfortunately, the bleeding was not due to hemorrhoids as he believed but an advanced inoperable colon cancer. He travelled to Mexico and Germany for fraudulent treatments and after spending thousands of dollars he died a slow, painful death in middle age. All because "they" were not going to do "that" to him! It was a tragedy that never should have happened as he had so much to live for, including wealth, for which he had worked hard, but seldom enjoyed.

All you have to do is look around you to see other disasters waiting to happen. Why are millions of apparently intelligent human beings still puffing on cigarettes? One wonders, are these people living on another planet? The scientific evidence is overwhelming that inhaling smoke and multiple carcinogens can result in cancer. We still have no way of preventing many malignancies but we can prevent most lung cancers by tossing cigarettes away. Besides, many of these smokers are smart enough to make millions yet dumb-witted about a cancer that kills millions. The list of needless premature deaths goes on and on.

Luckily I have so far escaped these medical disasters that should never happen by being prudent about lifestyle choices. But now, at 90 years of age, I and others know that my time on this planet is getting short, so I'm often asked, "How did you get there?"

One reader asks, "I like your way of speaking and getting the message across. You sure are witty and energetic. It does not sound like you're in a "Home." So what's the secret of your longevity? I'm sure other readers wouldn't mind knowing."

It's been said it's better to be lucky than good. I was lucky to inherit the longevity gene. This is the best start any parent can give. And I was lucky to have parents who taught me not to spend it foolishly by following a risky lifestyle.

I've been lucky to like what I do. At an early age I had a single-minded passion to be a doctor. Hell would have had to freeze over to stop me from accomplishing it. Being accepted at The

Harvard Medical School put the icing on the cake.

I've been lucky to inherit the gene of "thinness" which decreases the risk of obesity and its related problems, such as Type 2 diabetes. But I also step on the scale every day. My diet isn't perfect but it avoids excessive fats, sugar, processed flour, and it concentrates on fruits, some vegetables and fibre.

I've been lucky to have the privilege of not being forced to retire. My plan is to do this 10 years after I'm dead! Being inactive physically and mentally slowly kills people.

I had the lucky break of becoming a journalist. That allowed me to interview Nobel Prize winner Dr. Linus Pauling, among others. He believed humans need high doses of vitamin C and lysine to wipe out coronary death. I'm convinced that without this knowledge I would not have survived to this age. See my web site www.docgiff.com to see what other vitamins and minerals I take.

Early in my medical career I realized that Pogo was right when he said, "We have identified the enemy and the enemy is us." So I haven't succumbed to the North American habit of popping a pill for every ache and pain, thus causing liver and kidney damage. This household has never even had an over-the-counter painkiller or any cold remedies on its bathroom shelves. Rather, I've followed Sir William Osler's wise advice for treating a cold. You put your hat on the bedpost, go to bed, start sipping whiskey, and when you see two hats you stop. It was Osler's way of telling people they were over-medicating themselves with pills.

Fortunately, I realized that radiation therapy has been overused, so I have limited my radiation exposure to CT scans, chest and dental X-rays, unless absolutely needed. Nor do I believe in the current fad of cholesterol-lowering drugs. Rather, for 16 years I have used high doses of vitamin C and lysine to keep my arteries open.

I've followed Sir William Osler's advice that, "alcohol for the elderly is what milk is for the young." I believe, as we age, alcohol in moderation is possibly the best therapy invented. It lowers blood cholesterol, helps oil the blood, (decreasing the risk of blood clot) and is a great relaxant after a busy day.

I've never underestimated the value of laughter. A sense of humour never killed anyone. And it maintains your sanity when you see the lack of common sense in today's medicine, politics and financial matters.

Napoleon Bonaparte, when wondering who to promote to General in his army, once asked his officers, "Is he lucky?" In war or peace, Russian roulette often decides who reaches the senior years.

So has all this brought me to my 90th year? I'm not in a "home" yet, but I have no delusions about luck. Sooner or later, it gives out. As Stein's Law says, "If something can't go on forever it has to stop. It's just a matter of when." And Stein's Law always wins.

As for how I want life to end, I hope it ends suddenly. But more and more of us are coming to a slow, miserable, agonizing end. Due to an aging population many people are developing Alzheimer's and other degenerative diseases that make the end of life a living hell.

I recently read where an asinine Canadian judge and nursing home both refused to honour what any sane person would consider a reasonable Living Will. They rejected it, allowing the patient's suffering to continue. There should be a special place in hell for such judges. I'll tell you later in the book what I have done to avoid this and why we should all get "mad as hell."

Pitfalls of Lifestyle
Death in the Electronic Age, and Magic Underwear

Do you want to die at an early age? Not many would answer "Yes" to this question. But a report in the *Canadian Medical Association Journal* says early death is happening due to the effects of the electronic age. Fortunately, there is a solution. But are people willing to accept the advice? And what is magic underwear?

Dr. Kirsten Patrick, in an editorial in the CMAJ, paints a dismal picture of what is happening to those addicted to the pleasures of the electronic age.

Patrick says ownership of modern conveniences such as television, computers and cars has dramatically decreased the amount of time that we move. After all, we can now even shop without getting out of a chair. The result is an increase in the number of people who are obese and diabetic in low and middle-income countries. Earlier death is the payment.

Patrick reports that the Canada Fitness Survey involving 17,000 people also showed more sitting time increased the risk of death, particularly from cardiovascular disease.

A larger study of 222,497 Australians aged 45 and older proved that those who sat 8 to 11 hours a day had a 15 percent increase in overall mortality. For those who sat over 11 hours daily, there was a shocking 40 percent increased risk.

Dr. Scott A. Lear and colleagues also reported in the CMAJ that those who own a television, computer, and particularly a car, are more likely to develop obesity and Type 2 diabetes. And other studies indicate that obesity and Type 2 diabetes are world-wide problems. In other words everyone should get moving.

The fact that too much sitting is bad for you is not new. Years ago I reported an English study showing that those who drove London's two level buses were more likely to suffer a heart attack. The ticket collectors who had to walk up the stairs were less affected by coronary attack.

All this reminds me of an interesting study reported by Dr. James Levine, Professor of Nutrition at the Mayo Clinic. His unique experiment revealed why some people are thin, others obese, and what to do about it.

Levine gave 1000 extra calories a day above their normal caloric intake to a group of both thin people and obese people for six weeks to see what would happen. He also fitted them with "magic" underwear that monitored their every move. It was impossible for them to even scratch an ear without the magic underwear picking up the action.

It turned out that obese people moved two-an-a-half hours less every day. This also meant they burned 350 fewer calories daily which was stored as fat. So the secret is to keep moving, shopping until you drop, rising from your chair or tapping your toes to get rid of these excess calories.

Remember we cannot change our basal metabolic rate that accounts for 60 percent of our daily energy. We each use this amount of energy to keep our organs functioning. Then another 10 percent of calories to absorb, digest and store food. This leaves 30 percent that must be used up or stored as fat. So, is it off to the gym?

Levine claims that "Most people don't like going to the gym and some don't go even if they like it." Moreover, it takes 30 minutes on a bike to just burn up 100 calories.

He says the best approach is to get out of your comfortable chair. Moreover, he practices what he preaches by integrating walking into his work. For instance, he answers telephone calls and e-mails while walking on his treadmill and talks to people while exercising on a stepping device. Since there are no chairs in his office, he stands to work.

The Mayo Clinic shares his enthusiasm. It employs "Movologists" to design furniture and offices to force people to move. Its message to children and others is that their legs were designed for walking. I vividly recall that, while visiting Kenya, I did not see any obese children. They walked miles to school every day.

It's taken eons for the human body to develop to its present state. But nature did not design it to accommodate the amount of calories we consume, nor the inactivity. I realize no one's going to toss electronic hardware or furniture out the window. But the distressing news indicates that all studies show electronic devices are winning.

Years ago, after writing the column about the English bus drivers, I read about a Japanese study. Researchers reported that we should walk 10,000 steps daily to ensure good health. So I purchased a pedometer which showed I was walking 11,000 steps a day. I believe this is one of the reasons I have reached 90+. We all have two good legs. Use them. It's good medicine.

Pitfalls of Lifestyle
Why I'm Not a Teetotaler
Remember, Jesus Turned Water into Wine

In my medical practice, I've always believed that what was good for me as a doctor was also good for my patients. But my first word of advice, bold and underlined, was the word MODERATION in all things. Above all, in the use of alcohol.

Many years ago I shocked nurses when I wrote a post-operative prescription for a patient stating that "This patient may have her favourite alcoholic drink on the third post-operative day if she wishes to do so."

Why did I do it? Because patients often begin to worry about their recovery two to three days after surgery. The fact that I will allow them an alcoholic drink reassures them I must believe they are indeed on the road to recovery. Besides, hospital routine is boring, even depressing, and this decreases their anxiety in recuperation.

Years ago I also wrote that there should be an English-style pub in every Canadian chronic care hospital. Actually, there was one, the Boars' Head Pub at Sunnybrook Veterans Hospital in Toronto. I visited it to get a first-hand look at its care. The pub was serviced by a buxom bar maid who didn't have a degree in psychology. But she had more savvy than many doctors while helping to bring cheer into the lives of the chronically ill.

The pub's drawing force was not just beer. Some patients just wanted a soft drink or the opportunity to talk to others bored with the daily hospital routine. Patients were allowed two drinks of beer a day and the Royal Canadian Legion provided funds for what I believe was the only hospital pub in Canada or the U.S. Now it has regrettably closed and chronic care patients are once again looking at four bleak walls all day. Visit a chronic care facility and decide for yourself. Would you prefer a beer or your favourite alcoholic drink, or sedatives? I guess you know what my choice would be.

So my daily routine after a surgical morning and seeing patients in the afternoon was a 30 minute walk home, and an alcoholic beverage while watching the evening news. After all, the evening news is full of disaster, and a pre-dinner drink not only provided me with relaxation after a stressful day, but perspective as well.

Now having seen my last patient 3 years ago on my 87th birthday, my office is in a condo overlooking Lake Ontario. I spend my days writing, sometimes successfully and sometimes less so. For instance, if I've had a good writing day and believe my copy deserves the Nobel Prize in Literature, it's rewarding to end the day with my usual rum and Diet Coke. But if I end the day and believe everything I've written deserves to be tossed into the waste paper basket, I really, really need the comfort of a soothing beverage.

I realize that alcohol in excess is a huge personal and social problem. It causes health problems as well as chaos in society and on our roads. So if any reader is unable to use alcohol moderately they should not use it at all. But I would not want to return to the days of prohibition. After all, we don't ban the use of cars just because some idiot drives at excessive speeds.

Here are 10 reasons why I consider moderate drinking a healthy habit:

One – I enjoy life and want to live longer. The American Cancer Society recently studied the drinking habits of 500,000 Americans. They found that one alcoholic drink a day in middle age decreased the risk of premature death by 20 percent.

The reason is that alcohol contains antioxidants which eliminate free radicals, the waste products of metabolism, believed to be associated with aging, heart disease and cancer. And, by the way, if you like Martinis don't ignore James Bond's advice. He always orders "shaken" martinis. Now we know they contain more antioxidants than "stirred" martinis.

Two – Regular consumption of alcohol lowers the risk of heart attack by 30 to 50 percent! Alcohol dilates blood vessels and increases high density lipoprotein (HDL), the good cholesterol, which removes bad cholesterol from circulation. It also makes platelets more slippery, providing less chance of a blood clot in coronary arteries. And it lowers blood fibrinogen, a small particle that's part of the clotting process.

Three – Two recent studies show that light consumption of alcohol significantly decreases the risk of stroke, the type caused by a blood clot.

Four – Macular degeneration is the most common cause of blindness in people over age 65. It's now believed that alcohol reduces the risk of this disease. And it reduces the chance of arterial blockage in the lower legs.

Five – In 1998 France's National Institute of Health and Scientific Research reported an interesting finding. A study suggested that elderly people who drink moderate amounts of wine are less likely to suffer from senility and Alzheimer's Disease than teetotalers. Now, an 18 year old study of 3,500 Japanese Americans in Hawaii has more good news. Those who drank up to one alcoholic beverage a day were 40 percent less likely to have a poor score on cognitive brain function tests than non-drinkers. This finding is not surprising since autopsies on Alzheimer patients show microscopic areas of degeneration in the brain. This likely results from atherosclerosis in tiny arteries which decreases oxygen supply to the brain. Without sufficient oxygen brain cells die.

Six – Today, there's an unprecedented epidemic of Type 2 diabetes. Every 30 seconds a new diabetic is diagnosed in North America. The reason? Obesity. So one could argue the last thing obese people need is more calories from alcohol. But luckily alcohol increases the effectiveness of insulin. In effect, our cells become more responsive to insulin which lowers blood sugar.

Seven – Another disease, osteoporosis (brittle bones), affects large numbers of elderly people. The majority of fractured hips are due to this problem and their treatment costs our health care system millions of dollars. A Finnish study evaluated the bone density and alcohol consumption of 3,200 postmenopausal women for six years. The teetotalers lost a larger amount of bone.

Eight – I don't like the hypocrisy of doctors. At international medical meetings, numerous studies show moderate drinking helps longevity. But the majority of doctors refuse to tell patients about them because they will increase alcoholism, drunken driving and other social problems. I too condemn irresponsibility.

But isn't it dishonest to keep sensible people in the dark about the benefits of alcohol simply because some abuse it?

Nine – Don't forget the relaxing effects of alcohol in our over-stressed world.

Ten – I believe what some of the most brilliant minds have said about alcohol use. Hippocrates, the Father of Medicine, supported the medicinal use of alcohol. Sir William Osler the esteemed professor of medicine at McGill, Johns Hopkins and Oxford Universities claimed that "alcohol is for the elderly what milk is for the young." Add to this the wise counsel of Armand Cardinal Richelieu who remarked, "If God forbade drinking, would he have made wine so good?" And don't forget that Jesus supported the use of alcohol. After all, he transformed water into wine. So why would a lowly mortal like me want to ignore all these sage teachings? Particularly when there are more old wine drinkers than old doctors!

So what is moderate drinking? One or two drinks a day. (one drink equals 12 ounces of beer, 5 ounces of wine or one-and-a-half ounces of hard liquor). But if you've never touched a drop of alcohol or can't be a moderate drinker, forget everything I've said. I've no desire to add to our social problems!

Pitfalls of Lifestyle
90+ With All My Teeth

Over 400 years ago, Miguel de Cervantes, author of *Don Quixote*, realized the importance of sound teeth. Don Quixote said, "For I would have you know, Sancho, that a mouth without molars is like a mill without a stone, and a tooth is more precious than a diamond."

I've always believed Cervantes was way ahead of his time. This is why at 90+ I have not lost one tooth. Taking care of your teeth is not just a cosmetic issue. What goes on in the teeth and gums also affects other parts of the body.

Yet many people today don't appreciate the importance of Quixote's message. Today, tooth decay affects 96 percent of the population. Two out of five North Americans over age 19 have lost teeth. And over age 65 one in five have no teeth, often due to gum disease.

Dental rust, known as periodontal gum disease (PGD), is an insidious process. In its early stages the gum turns from a natural pink to red. Later, small spaces form between the gum and tooth. Called gingivitis, the condition is not usually painful and can remain unnoticed for many years.

However, gingivitis usually turns into periodontitis, and the gum starts to pull away from the crown and root of the tooth creating deep pockets in which bacteria accumulates. The end result is that the firm supporting structures of the teeth are destroyed.

To prevent PGD, people must get rid of common misconceptions. You have to do more than just see your dentist for regular checkups or brush your teeth. 90 percent of my patients believe that sound dental hygiene involves only brushing teeth after each meal.

Professor Giovanni of Padua University, Italy, preached the right idea in the 15th century. He said, "If all particles of food were removed from between the teeth after each meal and the mouth cleaned night and morning, care could be effective."

But it's possible to brush your teeth a dozen times after a meal without removing the food between teeth. To see the result, use dental floss or stimudents after eating blueberries or other food, to see how much food remains between teeth. This "no man's land" between teeth traps food, promotes infection, and destroys the tough periodontal fibres that cement the teeth in place.

But it's hard to get this hygienic message across to all ages. Years ago I flew onto the deck of the nuclear aircraft carrier, the USS Nimitz. This massive ship carries 6,000 sailors with an average age of 19. I was amazed to hear that seven dentists working day after day could not keep up with the dental decay of the crew.

People who get lazy about dental hygiene fail to realize the loss of a tooth means more than just the loss of a tooth. George Herbert, in 1640, wrote "For want of a nail the horse's shoe was lost. For want of a shoe the horse was lost. For want of a horse the rider was lost. For want of a rider the battle and the kingdom was lost." Lost teeth leave holes. Nothing supports opposing teeth while chewing. So they too become loose and more susceptible to decay.

I recently attended my Harvard Medical School Reunion in Boston and listened to a variety of professors discussing new advances in medicine. I learned that there may be an end to drilling and filling decay in teeth. Good news for those who fear the drill.

This research was reported in the Journal, *Science Translational Medicine*. David Mooney, a Harvard University bioengineer, says that shining a light from a low powered laser, about the brightness of a sunlit day, enabled the teeth to regrow dentine, the inner material that makes up the bulk of the tooth. So far this has been accomplished just in rodents.

But Harold Slavkin, a Professor of Dentistry at the University of California, says that this work in rodents sets the stage for dramatic changes in medical care. People in the future will be able to regrow their own teeth, hearts and other organs.

Before this happens Cervantes would tell you it's possible to keep your teeth a lifetime. Be sure to get regular dental checkups, keep a tooth brush at the office and stimudents in your pocket. And remember what Giovanni taught in the 15th century still applies today.

If you're still not convinced do the blueberry test and see firsthand that Giovanni was right. Then you will have all your teeth at 90+.

Pitfalls of Lifestyle

Why I Had More Energy Than My Father

So what else could be responsible for my reaching 90+? I often hear this remark from long-standing family friends, "You're so like your mother, you have so much energy!" I admit energy-wise they're right. My Father preferred to sit in his chair analyzing mathematical problems, while Mother had high octane gas. She never stopped running around. But I didn't know why I inherited her energy until I read a report in the *Nutrition Action Health Letter* about mitochondria. So, here's another reason for my longevity and how you can increase your energy level.

It's said that precious things come in small packages, and there's no better example than mitochondria. Each cell in our body contains up to 2,000 mitochondria and, although tiny, they make up to 60 percent of the volume of muscle cells and 40 percent of heart cells.

Simon Melov, Director of the Genomics Core at the Buck Institute for Age Research in California, reports that "mitochondria are the power plants of our cells, tiny furnaces within the cells of our body that burn food for energy."

But how does this make me like my mother? Yes, mitochondria have their own genetic material. But unlike the DNA in the cell's nucleus, which comes from both parents, mitochondria DNA is passed down from mother to child. This may be why

I've had the chance of living into my nineties, as did my mother.

Tory Hagen, a researcher at the Linus Pauling Institute, Corvallis, Oregon, says, "Mitochondria have been called the Achilles' heel of the cells in aging." Essentially, the healthier the mitochondria, the longer the life.

These tiny mitochondria furnaces are continually using oxygen to burn fat, protein and carbohydrates to generate energy. This oxidation process results in the formation of free radicals, metabolic ash that may also damage mitochondria.

Mark Mattson, chief of the Cellular and Molecular Neuroscience Section at The National Institute of Health, says weakened mitochondria may leave people susceptible to Parkinson's Disease or accelerate the downward trend of Alzheimer's Disease.

So how can you increase the number and strength of mitochondria? First, never forget the importance of exercise. David Hood, a researcher at York University in Toronto, says exercise can increase the number of mitochondria by 40 to 50 percent in six weeks. It's necessary to walk, run, bicycle or swim briskly for 20 minutes three to four times a week. You must continue these exercises to maintain healthy mitochondria and younger muscles.

In 2002, Dr. Bruce Ames, a researcher at the University of California, and his colleague Tory Hagan, made international headlines. They reported that old, sedentary rats (roughly equal to humans aged 70 to 100 years) perked up and "danced the Macarena" after being fed carnitine and lipoic acid. Lipoic acid is an antioxidant, and according to Hagen, carnitine pushes fat into mitochondria and gives a boost to their activity.

Ames and Hagen also discovered that rats given these two nutrients had less mitochondria damage in their brains. In beagle dogs, they increased short term memory.

A combination of carnitine and lipoic acid is available to consumers called Juvenon, and there is considerable information about it on the web site www.juvenon.com/info. The problem is this remedy is patented, not cheap, and only available by calling the toll-free number 1-800-309-0970.

I asked Dr. Andrew Weil, Professor of Integrative Medicine at the University of Arizona, if this study made any sense. Weil is an internationally recognized expert on alternative medicine. He's travelled widely to study medicinal plants in South America and Africa and has been a major proponent of omega-3 fatty acids, vitamin D and health benefits of fruits, vegetables and fish. He says that Juvenon is a remarkable health supplement and he takes it daily. But he neglected to say whether if makes him dance the Macarena!

So what's the message? Rats lacking the right nutrients get tired, don't want to run on a treadmill, nor swim too far, and cannot find cheese in a maze. Humans react the same way if they fall into the trap of consuming too many packaged foods laden with unhealthy ingredients. If that happens, mitochondria do not function efficiently. Adding a little carnitine and lipoic acid may prompt you too to start dancing the Macarena!

As for me, dancing was not one of the things that got me to 90+!

Pitfalls of Lifestyle

How I Escaped Another Big Killer

I was in my final year of surgical training at The Harvard Medical School when one of my students said to me. "For old times sake, you should come to the school dance at Vanderbilt Hall this Saturday night." He added, "Besides, my girl friend at Wellesley College has a classmate from Toronto who is going, and you must know her!" I advised my American student I did not know everyone in Canada. But for nostalgic reasons I decided to revisit my former medical residence. It was one of those lucky decisions because I met this attractive, intelligent Canadian girl from Toronto. And I immediately fell in love with her. We were soon married. I didn't know it then, but I know now she may have saved my life!

Now I wonder how I could have been so stupid. But years ago smoking cigarettes had not become the demon that we know today. Yet shortly after our marriage it became obvious that my wife disliked the habit. One day she said to me, "You should stop smoking." Stupidly, I asked "For how long?" She replied, "Forever!" To please her, I quit cold turkey.

Looking back, as a doctor, I should have made this decision myself. It's been said that, "If you keep going to hell, you will eventually get there." And I was headed in that direction. Today it's unbelievable that millions of North Americans are headed the same way in spite of concrete evidence that smoking kills. There are few greater examples of human madness.

Sir Walter Raleigh, a favourite courtier of Queen Elizabeth I, introduced tobacco to England. But if he tried this today, authorities would hang him for even suggesting its use. Tobacco would be banned as a hazardous substance. Now, we know tobacco contains 4,000 chemicals of which 40 are known to cause cancer in humans. It's ironic that no sane person would swallow a pill that has this lethal mixture, yet many willingly smoke cigarettes that contain it.

The facts are appalling. Every year tobacco kills at least three million people worldwide. Today 90 percent of lung cancer deaths, 30 percent of all cancers, 80 percent of chronic bronchitis and emphysema and 25 percent of heart disease and stroke are due to tobacco. Looking at these figures you might think that giving mouth to mouth resuscitation to Dracula was safer than lighting up a toxic cigarette.

I, along with some doctors, finally got the message. A generation ago 50 percent of doctors smoked. Today, just 7.9 percent of physicians smoke. We have seen the lungs of smokers who eventually need an oxygen tank to breathe, or suffer a slow painful death from lung cancer. However, since smoking can take 20 years or more to either kill or cause chronic disease, prevention has always been a hard sell.

Today, it appears that women are as foolish as men. More women have started smoking, and unfortunately are dying like men. It's a public health tragedy. Lung cancer has now surpassed breast cancer as the number one killer of women.

"Get your priorities straight," I've said to some patients. For instance, female patients often worry about the use of estrogen or the birth control pill. Yet they continue to suck in the poisonous vapors of cigarettes. These women who continue to smoke don't need me as a doctor, they require a psychiatrist.

To other die-hard smokers I've suggested. "Why don't you suck your thumb instead of smoking?" It's known that part of the rationale of smoking is the hand-to-mouth ritual. Studies show that smokers repeat this ritual 200 times a day or 73,000 times a year. That's a lot of ritual. It's one of the reasons so many types of treatment fail.

Several years ago during a trip to England I interviewed Richard Pito, Professor of Epidemiology at Oxford University. He reported that people who start smoking early in life decrease their longevity by 20 years.

Johnny Carson, the long-standing star of TV's "Tonight Show" was said to repeat over and over as he was slowly dying from emphysema, "Damn those cigarettes." He should have said it years earlier.

What is damnably frustrating are the multi-millionaire celebrities who are paid to be photographed smoking a cigarette or stogie. One hockey coach was photographed smoking a stogie. The next day his heart was being monitored due to shortness of breath. Yet the following day he was again caught smoking a stogie! The madness continues.

To debunk a myth, cigar smoking is not a safe alternative to cigarettes. Rather, a single stogie contains as much nicotine as a pack of cigarettes. Moreover, the smoke is more carcinogenic, containing over 60 known carcinogens. It also has more ammonia, tar and lethal gas, carbon monoxide. A single stogie emits 20 times the amount of carbon monoxide as a single cigarette.

We will never know how many deaths occur on our highways from this sleep-inducing poison. But we do know the numbers that die from cancer or other diseases such as emphysema.

What a lucky day for me when I decided to spend an evening at my former medical residence. I might never have met the no-

nonsense student from Toronto. If I had continued to smoke, I may never have reached 90+.

Pitfalls of Cardiovascular Disease

Linus Pauling Changed and Saved My Life

Would I be alive in 2014, following a heart attack over 16 years ago, if I had not interviewed Dr. Linus Pauling? I believe that answer is a thundering "No". It's been said that even the mangy street dog has his lucky days and I got lucky 25 years ago. I decided to interview Dr. Linus Pauling for a column during his visit to Toronto. The first thing he told me during my two hour interview was that animals manufacture vitamin C. Human he said, lost this ability eons ago due to genetic mutation. I found this fascinating because none of my esteemed professors had ever mentioned this to me during my time at The Harvard Medical School. But then I made a huge mistake. I did not take Pauling's advice and big doses of vitamin C. It nearly cost me my life in 1998.

On a beautiful Sunday morning, the sun was shining, the birds were singing and God was in Heaven. I was also very pleased with life as I was about to leave in seven days for Argentina to see my eldest son married. But within a few seconds I knew I wasn't going anywhere. I was having a heart attack. It was a severe attack and I nearly died in the next 24 hours. Luckily, with immediate care I survived and six weeks later had the good fortune to undergo a triple bypass operation done by Dr. Tirone David, a superb cardiac surgeon.

But then I had to make one of the biggest decisions of my life. My cardiologist said that, due to the severity of the heart attack and increased blood cholesterol, it was critical that I immediately start a cholesterol-lowering-drug (CLDs). Several other cardiologists in Canada and others I had met at international meetings in Europe all agreed it was utter madness if I did not take CLDs. They all stressed that numerous studies prove that CLDs are the be-all-and-end-all to treat the number one killer, heart disease. So criticizing the value of CLDs was like damning Motherhood and apple pie. It was a tough decision and I spent hours considering what to do. I had a wonderful wife, four great children and grandchildren and had no desire to leave this planet.

So the decision? At this point I had been a surgeon for many years and if that had been the complete story of my life, I'm 99.9 percent certain I would have readily agreed to CLDs. But I was aware from contact with many patients that this medication often resulted in unintended consequences, the possibility of liver, kidney, muscle pain and emotional problems and in some cases death.

But I had also been a syndicated medical journalist for 23 years and this had been a huge educational experience. I had, by this time, travelled the world and interviewed many international researchers, Linus Pauling being at the top of the list. In fact, prior to my heart attack, I had another two hour interview with this Nobel Prize winning scientist.

One other factor lead to my decision. I had never forgotten about Leonardo da Vinci. Five hundred years ago he wrote that "nature never breaks her own laws". In effect, he was saying "Don't mess around with nature" as it has taken eons for it to determine how much cholesterol, magnesium, and other ingredients our bodies need. History has shown that if you disregard this advice, there are always unintended consequences.

So I finally decided to bet my life on Linus Pauling. I believed his research more than I believed the money-driven research of pharmaceutical companies who were making billions of dollars on CLDs each year. It was a bit of a crap shoot because at that time I was not aware of other research that proved Pauling right. It was 13 years later that Dr. Sydney Bush, an English researcher proved that high doses of vitamin C and lysine could, not only prevent, but reverse atherosclerosis (hardening of arteries). This revolutionary discovery deserves the Nobel Prize and has had a profound effect on my life.

My obstinacy made me aware of how doctors react when you say "no" to their treatment. If you're not a medical doctor and don't take their advice, this quickly fractures what was previously a good relationship. But let me tell you something. Even if you are a doctor you still do not escape outright rejection. You realize quickly you no longer have a doctor. If I had been in this position I would have said, "Giff, I think you are a damn fool when all the scientific studies show you should take CLDs. But I will still be your doctor and eventually you will realize you have made the mistake of your life."

So for the moment I became my own doctor. I knew Pauling took 20,000 milligrams (mg) of vitamin C daily along with 5,000 mg of lysine. I decided to start with 10,000 of C and 5,000 of lysine in divided doses during the day. This required swallowing 30 tablets daily. I didn't like this but decided it was better than dying. I would still be taking these pills today, but once again I got lucky. I met Deane Parks, President of Preferred Nutrition. I complained about my routine of pill-taking. He remarked, "I believe we can make a powder of vitamin C and lysine. Four months later Medi-C Plus, the combination, was available in Health Food Stores in both powder and pill form.

What a difference! I now take scoops of Medi-C Plus mixed

with either water or orange juice. Or I sprinkle some on my morning cereal. Or at 5:00 o'clock I mix it with my pre-dinner drink, dark rum and Diet Coke.

Linus Pauling gave me these last 16 years.

Pitfalls of Cardiovascular Disease

EP=a2 Has Killed More People than E=mc2

It's been said Einstein's E=mc2 (energy=mass x C speed of light squared) is the world's most important scientific equation. Unfortunately it created the atomic bomb that killed thousands in World War II. But I believe my equation EP=a2 (extra pounds = atherosclerosis squared) is the world's important medical equation. Regrettably, it's killing more millions every year than E=mc2. Think again if you believe this is exaggerated.

Consider human obesity. Nothing, including the thousands of books on weight loss and diet, has been able to stop the epidemic of obesity which gets worse world-wide every year.

Nor does anyone have the solution to the problem of increasing numbers of people developing Type 2 diabetes. The U.S Centers for Disease Control and Prevention reports that one in 13 North Americans have diabetes. And one in four over the age of 65 suffers from this disease.

Then there are an estimated 14 million people in North America who don't even know they have diabetes!!!! And millions more have prediabetes, just one step away from diabetes and its complications. All these figures increase every year.

So how does this combination kill? It's because EP (extra pounds) = a2 (atherosclerosis), causes the rust that collects in all of our arteries as we age. We have known for years that people who are obese or have diabetes (or both) always develop more of this deadly rust that is composed of fatty deposits and cholesterol.

The deadly trio of obesity, diabetes and heart attack will eventually bring our health care system to its knees. Years ago this scenario was rare. More people died from infection. Now, since we live longer, the *Gifford-Jones Law* has a major effect on longevity with development of degenerative diseases. *Gifford-Jones Law* states that one disease often leads to another, and another. The best example is that obesity leads to Type 2 diabetes and 50 percent of diabetics die of a heart attack due to atherosclerosis.

The problem isn't complicated. If all the toilets in the country stopped flushing due to plugged pipes, civilization as we know it would quickly end. If the organs of our body lack oxygenated blood due to plugged arteries, our own lives on this planet end.

It's been said that you can whip a tired horse only so long before it drops. Extra pounds similarly put tremendous stress on the pancreas. It eventually collapses and stops producing insulin.

When I graduated from The Harvard Medical School 65 years ago only 5 percent of people had Type 2 diabetes and 95 percent was due to genetics. Now, 95 percent develop Type 2 diabetes (better called lifestyle diabetes) due to obesity, and obese children usually become obese adults. This means they face the increased risk of blindness, kidney failure, leg amputation and heart attack.

Atherosclerosis is therefore the ultimate destroyer, gradually decreasing the amount of oxygenated blood and other nutrients that are necessary for all organs. Just as a car cannot run without gas, the pancreas and other organs falter without oxygen.

So what is going to happen in the future? The answer is that EP=a2 will continue to kill more than Einstein's equation. The blunt truth is that only draconian measures by government and citizens will stem the epidemic of obesity and Type 2 diabetes. Hell will freeze over before that happens.

But there is a simple, natural way to put a dent in the progress of the nation's number one killer, heart attack. Research shows that high concentrations of vitamin C and lysine, readily available as Medi-C Plus in Health Food Stores and select natural pharmacies, can reverse atherosclerosis. It's a revolutionary discovery that deserves the Nobel Prize. But it's a national tragedy that this research is collecting dust and is being ignored by the medical establishment, particularly cardiologists who should be aware of it.

Why have I been able to reach 90+ without EP=a2 killing me? There's no doubt heredity played a role. But I've also stepped on the scale every day to make sure I'm not getting obese. That's helped me circumvent Type 2 diabetes and the big killer atherosclerosis. And for 16 years a day never goes by without me taking high doses of vitamin C and lysine.

See the web site www.docgiff.com to see the dramatic changes of arteries treated by vitamin C and lysine. You don't have to be a cardiologist to see the striking difference. If only cardiologists would look at what is so obvious!

Pitfalls of Cardiovascular Disease

Can Vitamin C Stop an Aging brain?

"I want to die with my boots on" is an often used expression. But that poses a problem. Today, many are living and dying not even knowing their boots are on.

Does Alzheimer's Disease (AD) have to happen? Are cholesterol deposits in arteries starving our brain cells of oxygen? I've been taking high doses of vitamin C and lysine for over 16 years hoping this may save me from dementia and Alzheimer's Disease.

A report in the journal, *Dementia and Geriatric Disorders*, claims there's a link between heart attack and Alzheimer's Disease. The link is atherosclerosis (hardening of arteries) due to cholesterol.

Sir William Osler, Professor of Medicine at both McGill and Johns Hopkins Universities, once remarked that "it's lucky to be born with good rubber." Namely, it's best to have flexible, open arteries that carry sufficient amounts of oxygenated blood to the body's organs. After all, we know what happens in a house with clogged pipes. In humans, narrowed, cholesterol laden arteries cause the same collapse.

Researchers at the Kaiser Permanente Center in Oakland, California, and the University of Kuopio in Finland, followed 10,000 people for 40 years. They found that high blood cholesterol was associated with a 66 percent higher risk of AD. Moreover, those with even borderline levels of blood cholesterol were 52 percent more likely to develop this frightening disease.

The brains of people with Alzheimer's Disease contain lumps of what's called amyloid plaques. They cause nerve cell death in the brain, and the first to be attacked are the nerves in the brain's memory center.

Researchers at Lund University in Sweden discovered that when they treated the brain tissue of mice suffering from AD with vitamin C, the amyloid plaques dissolved.

What causes AD and how to treat this crippling disorder is still unknown. But I'd agree with Osler that open, flexible arteries are the prerequisite to good health. And vitamin C, a powerful antioxidant, is known to rid the body of free radicals, end products of metabolism.

But what is the relationship between the heart and Alzheimer's Disease? We know that coronary arteries, clogged with cholesterol deposits, make heart attack the number one killer. We also now know something we did not know until a few years ago, that high concentrations of vitamin C and lysine can reverse atherosclerosis lesions in coronary arteries. This is a discovery of unparalleled proportions and photographic evidence proves it happens.

Dr. Alvaro Alonso, Assistant Professor of Epidemiology at the University of Minnesota's School of Public Health, reports that post-mortem studies reveal that the brains of patients suffering from dementia often show damage to small arteries. These arteries may have triggered small strokes that eventually lead to brain damage.

The last thing we need as we age is intracranial atherosclerosis that triggers small areas of brain damage. So is vitamin C able to prevent it?

Other studies I found in medical literature claimed that vitamin C was either controversial or had been shown to be ineffective in treating Alzheimer's Disease. But these studies have one monumental flaw. Researchers were using no more than 500 milligrams (mgs) of vitamin C daily, a totally ineffective dose.

These results reminded me of the Harvard study that claimed vitamin C had no effect on coronary disease. How could it be? They were using only 75 mgs of C! As Linus Pauling used to tell his critics, "It's the dosage, stupid".

I do not possess a crystal ball, nor am I related to the Almighty. But old- fashioned horse sense tells me that, since a product called Medi-C Plus contains 6,000 mgs of vitamin C and 3,900 mgs of lysine, and can prevent and reverse cholesterol blockages in coronary arteries, it can also do the same to arteries in the brain.

But hell will freeze over before an expensive study using high amounts of C and lysine is done. These ingredients cannot be patented so who would pay for it? In the meantime, those who are already taking high doses of C and lysine for cardiac reasons, will hopefully get the added benefit of decreasing the risk of developing AD.

Pitfalls of Cardiovascular Disease

Cardiologists Should Consult an Eye Doctor

Oliver Cromwell, The Lord Protector of England, on August 3rd, 1650, lashed out at his critics in parliament saying, " I beseech you in the bowels of Christ, think it possible you may be mistaken?"

During the past year I have shared Cromwell's frustration. I have been trying to convince doctors, particularly cardiologists and health officials, that high doses of vitamin C and lysine could save millions of North Americans from heart attack and other cardiovascular problems. In addition, save millions of dollars for our health care system.

But what has happened? To put it bluntly, I may as well have been talking to the moon as far as doctors are concerned. I've written several columns about the health benefits of C and Lysine, been interviewed on radio and TV, and travelled to most parts of Canada speaking about this therapy. I have not been speaking about old-fashioned snake oil. Rather, I've been presenting scientific proof that this natural remedy can not only prevent atherosclerosis (hardening of arteries), but also reverse this lethal disease. It's been 65 years since I graduated from The Harvard Medical School and I believe this is the most revolutionary discovery that has happened since that time.

I realize that some would counter, "What about new operations giving people new hips and knees?" These procedures are great technical achievements. However, a surgical operation does not cure the arthritis that required the operation. On the other hand, high doses of C and lysine reverses atherosclerosis, the rust inside arteries that robs the organs of oxygenated blood, and triggers so many cardiovascular complications.

Luckily, thousands of health-conscious people have listened to the evidence. They believe the science makes sense. But doctors have been conspicuously absent. I realize that doctors are busy, but one would think that some physicians, particularly cardiologists, would be curious about this research. Moreover, there's been no e-mail complaints about Medi-C Plus, or any challenge from the medical profession, health organizations or Ministers of Health in any of the Canadian Provinces. So why is the profession so silent? It's strange because when I have been involved in previous medical controversies, they have triggered a massive response from the medical establishment. Could it be that it has no ammunition to fire?

What I find particularly distressing is that this research is not the usual statistical study, subject to the criticism that "there are three kinds of lies, lies, damn lies and statistics." Rather, vitamin C research is backed by the expertise of Dr. Linus Pauling, a Nobel Prize winner, a New Zealand pathologist, and an English researcher who, for the first time in history, has photos to prove this treatment is effective

This is why I believe that cardiologists should consult with their eye doctor if they cannot see the difference between "before and after" photos of patients' retinas treated with high C and lysine. The difference is so obvious that a young child could see the disparity in the retinal photos. And since the head is connected to the body, common sense dictates that these same changes are occurring in coronary and other arteries.

The medical establishment always insists that double blind studies must be carried out using high doses of vitamin C and lysine. But this will never be done as vitamin C and lysine are natural remedies that cannot be patented. So what company will spend tens of millions of dollars doing these studies with no chance of reaping a profit? Besides, double-blind studies with one group of volunteers receiving medication and the others getting a placebo leave much to be desired. In fact, the Bush photos are worth more than a thousand double blind statistical studies. Photos don't lie.

There may be several reasons why the medical establishment casts a blind eye at this natural remedy. They have been brainwashed by the hundreds of millions advertising dollars spent by big pharma on CLDs, touted as the be-all-and-end-all treatment of heart disease. Criticizing CLDs is like bashing the virtues of motherhood and apple pie.

Historically, there's also long convincing evidence that new medical ideas are not easily accepted by doctors. For instance, when Dr. James Linde, a British naval surgeon, showed that lime juice cured scurvy in sailors on long sea voyages it took 60 more years before this life-saving juice was accepted by the naval bureaucracy in London. Another classic example is when Dr. Semmelweiss, a professor at the University of Vienna, showed that by washing his hands following an autopsy, women in labour could be saved from dying of infection. Yet he was ridiculed by his colleagues, driven off the hospital staff, and died in an insane asylum in Vienna.

Closed minds are still causing trouble in our so-called enlightened age. In 2012 Allan Smith, a New Zealand farmer, went fishing. On his return he became acutely ill and laboratory studies confirmed he had contacted the swine flu virus. Smith was given every antibiotic in the book, but became unconscious and eventually required life support. Doctors told the family there was no hope and advised pulling the plug.

A family member had read about Linus Pauling and how large doses of intravenous vitamin C could cure viral diseases. But when this was requested, doctors refused, saying it was not part of the protocol to treat swine flu and that vitamin C was worthless. It was only when the family arrived at the hospital with a lawyer who bluntly told the doctors that they and the hospital would be sued unless intravenous vitamin C was given. Faced with this choice doctors administered 500,000 milligrams the first day. This, along with additional vitamin C, resulted in a dramatic recovery. The lungs were cleared of fluid, Allan Smith became conscious and life-support was discontinued. Smith is alive and well.

The next chapter of this remarkable recovery is hard to believe. His doctors stressed, during a television interview, that Allan Smith's recovery was due to their antibiotics finally working! If modern-day doctors cannot link and accept this dramatic recovery to vitamin C, it's not surprising that they cannot accept a less sensational one, coronary atherosclerosis, which kills over a period of years. This attitude has allowed millions of people to die. It's going to kill more people in the future. The irony is it will also kill cardiologists and other doctors who are too blind to accept these scientific facts.

The ancient romans had a dictum: "Credite Rebus" – Believe the Facts. Surely it's reasonable to ask cardiologists to take a look at the facts and ask, "is it possible we may be mistaken about the benefits of cholesterol lowering drugs?"

Pitfalls of Obesity

Avoiding Obesity Got Me to 90+

For me, getting to 90+ is the result of many factors and one of the most important has been maintaining a normal weight. Some people might say I'm compulsive about weight. Why? It's because I step on the bathroom scale every morning. Others who dine with me say I'm the last person who should talk about obesity and what to eat. I like roast beef and creamy mashed potatoes. I also eat French fries and enjoy ice cream. And as you have already read, I enjoy a rum and diet cola most every night before dinner. So my diet is far from ideal. But I got to 90+ on this routine and have remained the same weight as I was decades ago. Part of my secret has been moderation. I don't indulge in ice cream or French fries every day.

Some patients have said to me "I never get on the scale. I know I'm gaining weight when my clothes become tight." The problem is that by that time, they've gained 30 pounds! Sorry, the scale may depress you, but it does not lie and the best way to increase the chance of living longer, to enjoy your hard earned money, is to step on the scale. This means that if you see a three pound increase after indulging on a weekend, you immediately take off those pounds by decreasing calories. Sorry, again. Don't believe anyone who says that calories don't count.

The maintenance of normal weight is a major step in avoiding the "deadly trio" of obesity, Type 2 diabetes and heart attack. These three prematurely end the lives of many North Americans.

Pitfalls of Obesity

The Battleship King George V and the Importance of Fibre

But there's more to keeping your weight under control than stepping on a scale.

Recently, a patient who is extremely health conscious asked, "If you had to pick the most important food, what would you choose?" I replied, "fibre". I've believed for years that fibre is the corner stone of a healthy diet and without adequate amounts people are headed to a variety of health problems.

The National Academy's Institute of Medicine formulates dietary recommendations for the government. It recently reported that the average North American consumes only 14 to 15 grams of fibre a day. This is a failing grade as it's less than half of what people should be eating.

Fibre's primary benefit never crosses the minds of most people. Fibre is bulky and therefore filling. Years ago, my father-in-law called it "roughage" and swore by it. You can drink a cola loaded with eight teaspoons of sugar, but it has practically no effect on deadening the hunger reflex. However, eat one apple containing 3.3 grams of fibre and you rarely need a second. The consumption of fibre is, therefore, one of the first steps to controlling weight.

This fact isn't rocket science or anything new. Medical history has reported the benefits of fibre for years. Dr. Denis Burkitt, a

British researcher, showed that African natives who consumed large amounts of fibre did not suffer from constipation, appendicitis or large bowel problems.

During the war between Britain and France in the 18th century food was scarce. The British parliament passed a law designed to stretch the supply of grain. This meant that 80,000 English soldiers ate bread from unbolted flour. Army physicians soon noted that the health of the troops improved.

Historians and those who are 90 + remember the Battleship King George V for chasing Germany's battleship, the Bismarck. But the history books fail to mention that constipation was rampant among the sailors. Their ship's surgeon Captain T. L. Cleave was also constipated and he hated to take laxatives. Faced with this situation Cleave decided to experiment on himself. For several days he consumed raw unprocessed bran. It cured his, and his sailors', constipation.

All these people were doing was what Hippocrates had preached in 400 BC. But as has been aptly said, "The only thing we learn from history is that we don't learn from history". Hippocrates' sage advice to the citizens of Athens was to keep healthy they must always have bulky bowel movements. He suggested they consume whole bread, fruits and vegetables.

In my office I knew immediately when patients were getting sufficient fibre. During rectal examination those with insufficient dietary fibre have small hard stools. Those eating large amounts of fibre have large, bulky stools as soft as toothpaste.

The best way to start the day is with a high fibre cereal. It's hard to beat All-Bran. Just one-third of a cup contains 10 grams of fibre. It would take nearly 4 cups of Cheerios to get the same amount of fibre!

High fibre bread is hard to find. Don't be fooled by labels. Look for the words "whole wheat" with two grams of fibre per slice. Those labeled "multigrain" or "wheat" may contain little or no fibre.

To boost fibre content further add lentils, black beans, green peas, pears, bananas, prunes, broccoli, tomatoes, celery and roasted almonds to your diet. Fibre supplements can be taken but it's better to obtain fibre from food.

I've suggested in my column that fibre reduces constipation but may also decrease the risk of colon cancer. Foods remaining in the bowel contain cancer-containing compounds. The longer food is left in contact with the intestinal wall, the greater the chance of malignancy. Some recent studies question this theory, but residue is rarely beneficial.

No one has ever proven that fibre is bad for you. But it's best to add it to the diet slowly as it may cause bloating and gas. Is there any way you can visibly see if you're eating enough fibre? Several years ago I suggested that you just had to look into the toilet bowl. If your stools seldom float, there's a good chance you are not getting sufficient fibre. But friends complained to me they suffered a stiff neck from this gymnastic!

What happened to Captain Cleave? He should have been awarded a Nobel Prize. But he became known as "The Bran Man" and the subject of ridicule. Another example of how a healthy discovery collects dust.

Pitfalls of Obesity

How PGX Fights Obesity

Unfortunately history shows that North Americans love to eat, and have difficulty increasing the amount of fibre in their diet. The end result is too many calories. It's a no-brainer that obesity wins the game. So, if your psyche is unable to push you away from the table and also unable to accept a healthy, but uninteresting fibre cereal, what can you do?

Fortunately, there's a natural, safe remedy called PGX that acts in the same way as a bland cereal. Both attack obesity by what's called "filling volume". In effect PGX makes the stomach feel full and diminishes the hunger reflex. PGX is no ordinary fibre. Rather PGX (PolyGlycopleX) is a super fibre that replaces the fibre you should be eating. This complex of natural polysaccharides has been reported in several medical journals and gram for gram provides more punch that any other fibre.

You don't have to be a nuclear physicist to understand the result. The soft gels when swallowed with a glass of water expand due to their ability to absorb many times their weight in water. This paralyses the hunger reflex by telling the brain the stomach is full. Eureka! No desire for a second helping. In fact, due to its multiple benefits some authorities have called PGX the "Holy Grail" to fight obesity.

There are more benefits. Studies show that PGX decreases cholesterol by 17 percent and helps to lower triglycerides. It also fights constipation by absorbing large amounts of water.

But I stress to patients that the biggest benefit is that by attacking obesity it also decreases the risk of Type 2 diabetes, another major killer. PGX slows down the digestion of food and maintains a more normal blood sugar level. This places less stress on the hormone, insulin, which regulates blood sugar. So there's less risk that an overworked pancreas becomes exhausted, resulting in diabetes and all its complications. You don't reach 90+ that way.

The dosage of PGX to start with is one to two softgels before meals with a glass of water and gradually work up to 3 to 6. This creates the same effect on the hunger reflex as three bowls of oatmeal! It's advisable to increase the dose gradually over several days. Taking too much may cause bloating and loose stools. You can also take 2.5 grams of granules with water or add to moist foods.

If you are taking medication be sure to take it one hour before PGX, or two to three hours after it, as it can slow the absorption of drugs.

So PGX is therefore a sound natural remedy to "fibreize" your diet along with following a healthy lifestyle. Never forget Pogo, the cartoon character, who stressed that, "We have identified the enemy and the enemy is us".

Pitfalls of Obesity
Can Humans Get Smart or Do We Need a Famine?

A U.S., radio interviewer recently asked me, "How can the obesity problem be solved in our country?" He expected me to discuss diets and other ways to fight this epidemic. But I surprised him by saying, "It would take a famine, unless people changed their ways." I really wanted to get the point across that obesity and its complications will bring that nation's healthcare system to its knees unless there is a draconian change in North American habits. Was my remark so startling? Not if you consider what health authorities are reporting.

For instance, a report from the Institute of Medicine in the U.S. says that nine million children older than six years of age are obese. Another U.S. report shows that children whose mothers are obese are 15x more likely to be obese by six years of age. We know from experience that obese children usually grow up to be obese adults. Canada is not immune to this problem.

Dr. Peter Nieman, Founder of the Pediatric Obesity Clinic in Calgary, reports that one in three children in Canada are overweight and developing adult diseases. It's appalling that he is seeing non-alcoholic fatty degeneration of the liver in kids. In the worst cases the child's liver ends up looking like the liver of those suffering from alcoholic cirrhosis!

Dr. Adriel Feldstein, a pediatric gastroenterologist at the Mayo

Clinic in Rochester, Minnesota, reports a similar story. Every week he sees several children with an average age of 12 who have symptoms of liver disease.

A recent report from the Centers for Disease Control in the U.S. says that one in 13 North Americans have diabetes. For those 65 years of age and over one in four has this disease. It's an appalling situation.

Pitfalls of Obesity

Even Immigrating to the U.S. is Dangerous

U.S. citizenship has many advantages. Its pledge of "Life, Liberty and the Pursuit of Happiness" being one of them. But there's a price to pay. Reports show that newcomers quickly adopt U.S. eating habits, gain weight and suffer from degenerative diseases. A German proverb says, "Abundance kills more than hunger." There is simply too much abundance of the wrong foods in North America. Supermarkets are full of things you should not eat or at least eat in moderation. But hell will freeze over before supermarkets remove these foods.

It's obvious in many grocery stores that consumers have not seen the tragedy of excessive weight. Fast foods loaded with sugar, salt and calories have become ingrained in their habits. Not many grocery carts today would pass the healthy food test. I believe it would take the coming of a Messiah to stop what is happening.

Restaurants don't help. Particularly in the U.S., every meal is supersize. Or it's Friday and "all-you-can-eat-night." Temptation is everywhere and it is not going to change. It comes at a price.

A study of Latino immigrants showed that 11 percent of their children show thickening of the carotid arteries due to atherosclerosis. This has never been previously seen at this age. These children with partially blocked arteries in the neck are well on their way to blocked coronary arteries and premature death.

What are doctors doing about this? Mostly they spend more time talking about the dangers of cholesterol than obesity. Yet more of their patients will die of the deadly trio, obesity, Type 2 diabetes and heart attack than succumb to elevated cholesterol. Even doctors cannot get their priorities straight.

So am I too far off track by suggesting it may take a famine to solve the obesity epidemic? It required the huge "Manhattan Project" to build the atomic bomb that killed thousands. Maybe we need another Manhattan Project to save millions destined to die of obesity and its multiple complications.

Pitfalls of Obesity

What You Can Learn from a Jockey

There is always hope. I well remember one patient in my office who took this matter into her own hands. The first thing she said to me was, "Do you want to see a picture of me taken two years ago?" I was of course curious and said, "Yes". I was surprised to see a photo of a plump 200 pound woman. She was now half that size. So I asked the obvious question, "How did you do it?" She replied she had always had a burning desire to be a jockey. The next day she would indeed ride a race horse.

Motivation was a huge factor in her success. She had learned that she would have to step on a scale every day to follow her progress and on a scale before every race. There's no doubt she had learned how to count calories whether they came from fat, protein or carbohydrates. This jockey knew that most people need only 1,700 to 2,000 calories daily and acted accordingly.

She described how she became an expert in reading the calories in packaged foods and how to avoid them. For instance, she never ate a pepperoni thick-crusted pizza. It contains 2,288 calories. Even one slice has 280 calories.

She also knew how to do the math, that 3,500 calories equal one pound of fat. So she started eating 500 fewer calories a day which means in one week she had lost one pound, on her way to a whopping 52 pounds the first year. In the next year she lost another 52 pounds.

She also showed me her calorie book which listed the foods she would never eat: two scoops of chocolate ice cream, 570 calories, a bagel with two teaspoons of cream cheese 450, a Big Mac hamburger 540, a Burger King Double Whopper 1,060, and a toasted tuna melt sub, 1230 (to name a few). By eating an orange rather than drinking a glass of orange juice she saved 50 calories. A teaspoon of mustard on a cheese sandwich instead of mayonnaise saved 100 calories. Substituting fruit for a muffin saved 350. Water, she said, became routine rather than sugary drinks and she had learned to enjoy coffee without cream.

She had also kept herself in good shape during the next two years by exercising. She had followed Abraham Lincoln's advice that we have two good doctors in our own body, our left and right leg. So she would take long walks in the morning and evening.

She had also followed the advice of the Earl of Derby who counselled, "If you can't find time for wellness, you will eventually have to find time for sickness."

Motivation was the key to success in losing weight and becoming a jockey. But how many obese people have such an overwhelming desire to lose weight? Studies show that the failure rate is about 95 percent. It's a dismal batting average and one reason PGX is not going out of business soon.

Pitfalls of Surgery

Is Your Parent Healthy Enough for Surgery?

Warren Buffett, believed to be the world's greatest investor, says, "Risk comes from not knowing what you're doing." Risk in surgery also comes from not knowing what you're doing. But in this case rather than losing your money you can lose your life. So, how does the fragility test save lives?

A report from Johns Hopkins University says that "50 percent of people over 65 will undergo surgery." It's therefore a forgone conclusion that the children of aging parents and their children will be asking, "Do you believe he or she is well enough to undergo an operation?"

Sometimes the answer is as easy as falling off a log. The parent simply does not need surgery. After all, why subject a 70 year old parent with only mild discomfort, that's not life-threatening, to a major operation? The benefit does not warrant the operative risk.

But suppose an elderly parent's quality of life is severely affected? How then do you assess the risk of surgery? In the past there have been several ways to evaluate it.

The "Lee Cardiac Index" looks at the possibility of cardiovascular problems based on the type of operation, the degree of cardiovascular disease, whether the patient suffers from diabetes, and how good kidney function is.

There's also a tool used by the American Society of Anesthesi-

ologists, called the "ASA score". Anesthetists and surgeons esti-
mate the patient's health using a scale of one to five. A score of
one says that in all probability the patient is fit for the operation.
A score of five indicates an unfit patient who is unlikely to survive surgery.

But it's been long recognized that some patients with a score
of one may do poorly and those with a score of five may thrive
after surgery. So these tests are unreliable and may be little better
than tossing a coin.

Dr. Linda Fried, founder of the Johns Hopkins Center on Aging and Health, has been working on this dilemma for 10 years.
She says that 20 percent of those over 80 are frail. Women more
so than men, because they start life with less muscle. Sometimes
their fragility results from a triggering event such as a sudden
illness or injury that leads to a loss of appetite, weight loss and
muscle mass. Or more often it's a combination of the ravages
of time along with decreased physical activity that decimates
muscle mass.

Her research has developed what's called the "Fragility Test"
which evaluates five aspects of the patient's health. If an elderly
person suffers from two or more of the following problems they
must be classified as frail.

First, unintentional weight loss of 10 pounds or more in the
last year accompanied by loss of muscle mass, called "sarcopenia".
Second, weakness demonstrated by poor grip strength. Three, an
exhausted feeling causing the remark "I feel I cannot get going
most days of the week". Four, less physical activity where they're
only using 2,700 to 3,380 calories for the entire week (compared
to a need of 1,600 calories a day). Five, a slow walking speed in
which men over 5 feet seven inches and women over five feet
three inches take seven or more seconds to walk 15 feet.

To test the accuracy of the fragility test, Hopkins researchers assessed 564 patients 65 years of age or older before they under-went major surgery. Prior to their operation they were classi-fied by the fragility test as either "frail", "moderately frail" or "not frail".

The results were published in the *Journal of the American Col-lege of Surgeons*. It showed that the moderately frail and the frail were twice as likely to suffer post-operative complications such as infection, respiratory distress or poor wound healing. The moderately frail were also 3x more likely and the frail 20x more likely to require a nursing home when they were discharged from hospital. Add it all up and the fragility test makes sense.

I used to judge the elderly patient another way. I've seen tough elderly patients who do better post-operatively than younger ones. These elderly have that look in their eye that tells you they still enjoy life, get out of bed with a purpose, see the glass still half-full, are willing to take a small risk to improve their quality of life, and are still trying to keep their body in shape. Surgery was a benefit to them. For the indolent, less so. (I do not con-sider myself indolent).

The moral? It's said that: "The race is not to the swift nor the battle to the strong." But if you're a gambler, that's where you put your money. So keeping mind and body in good shape certainly improves survival after surgery.

Pitfalls of Surgery
Minor Surgery
and the Holiday Inn

What has the Holiday Inn to do with surgery? During my years of teaching young surgeons I often reminded them of the advertising slogan of this hotel chain, "There are no surprises at the Holiday Inn." But one could never provide the same assurance to patients scheduled for surgery, even so-called minor surgery. Or as Harvey Cushing, professor of neurosurgery at The Harvard Medical School remarked, "There is no such thing as minor surgery. But there are a lot of minor surgeons."

Joan Rivers, the comedian, who had numerous cosmetic operations recently had her last one. Reports indicate it was a minor procedure, but ended in a cardiac arrest and death. She would have been safer spending the night at the Holiday Inn!

One patient who wrote to me said, "I like to skip for exercise, but one morning I slipped and broke my little toe. Several months later the toe rode up over the next one and I was referred to a surgeon." The surgeon said, "the problem is a minor one easily corrected by Mickey Mouse surgery!"

What followed was a series of unpleasant jolts. The patient expected to quickly return to work, but was surprised to see a big bandage on her foot. While watching the surgeon change the bandage she noticed the words "congenital deformity" on her medical chart. She was then surprised to see a large incision extending up her instep and equally upset on discovering part of the toe had been removed.

The surgeon also suffered a jolt when the patient angrily questioned him about the congenital deformity, saying, "I just broke my toe." The surgeon, who had failed to read the medical report of a broken her toe replied, " I don't know why you're fussing. You don't need little toes anyway."

But this was not the end of her troubles. The toe failed to heal and she was referred to another surgeon who did another "minor" operation. This was followed by a crippling post-operative stroke.

So you can be sure of the Holiday Inn, but never of minor surgery. We never know what fate lies in store for us. Post-surgical complications can include infection that fails to respond to antibiotics, continuing pain from the incision or a pulmonary embolism, the result of inactivity, that kills you. Another unsuspected case was that of Julie Andrews, the star of "The Sound of Music", who had a small polyp removed from her vocal cord. To her distress, she never sang again as well as before the surgery.

The moral of the story is never, never assume that minor surgery means zero complications. You won't fall into this trap if you ask the surgeon how long you will be in hospital and what risks are involved. It's also important to enquire what will happen if you decide not to have the operation.

For years I've stressed in my column that whether it's a minor or major operation you should go into surgery on a first-class ticket. I've spent most of my life as a surgeon and know that even the top technical surgeons can't guarantee the outcome. But good hands always get better results.

Finding good hands is easier said than done, particularly if you've moved to a new location. A good start is to avoid the game of Russian Roulette by taking the advice of a friend or golfing partner, as it may be right or very wrong. The president of the company may have the wrong surgeon.

The only people who know who is the better qualified surgeon are those who are intimately involved in the operating room. This means anesthetists and scrub nurses who see the surgeon operating day after day. So if you're lucky enough to know one through contact with friends, take their advice.

I've reached 90+ in spite of two major operations, in part because I knew who had the best hands. Fortunately, they also had warm personalities. But remember, if you're told Dr. X is the best surgeon, but has the bed-side personality of Dracula, don't look for another surgeon. It's the hands that are about to cure your problem, not his or her personality.

Pitfalls of Surgery
How I Was Saved from a Common Operation

To ask what goes on at The Shouldice Hospital is like asking, "Is the Pope Catholic?" This hospital situated in Thornhill, near Toronto, is a world-famous center for the repair of hernias. But is its reputation as good as they say? If so, why? And why is it possible for surgeons to repair one hernia and miss another one? To find the answers, I observed surgeons at Shouldice performing one hernia operation after another. So how did this save me from this type of surgery?

A hernia is a protrusion of bowel through the abdominal wall. There are various types of hernias, but there's no such thing as sexual equality in this condition. 90 percent occur in men.

The Shouldice success rate is outstanding, virtually 100 percent if there's been no previous surgery, and 98 percent if it's a repeat operation. The recurrence rate in other hospitals is 10 percent or more.

So what's the secret of Shouldice's success? First, its surgeons are excellent technicians. Good hands mean precise, speedy surgery. Then, the old story that "practice makes perfect", whether you're a plumber or a surgeon, increases the odds. Every day 35 hernias are repaired at the Shouldice Hospital. Talent and practice are a tough combination to beat.

Some patients are surprised that 96 percent of the time only local anesthesia is used at Shouldice for this 45 minute procedure. That's because it works well and is less risky since many elderly patients are also suffering from cardiac irregularities, hypertension, heart failure, are on anticoagulant therapy, or have had a previous heart attack.

Local anesthesia, along with Valium and a painkiller allow the majority of patients to walk away from the operating table. The result speaks for itself. During the last 55 years, 290,000 hernia operations have been performed at the Shouldice with only one in 10,000 deaths within 28 days of surgery.

Recovery time is short. Patients leave the hospital in two days and return to work usually within eight days. In fact, the recovery time of one male patient could surely enter the *Guinness Book of Records.*

One of the surgeons told me that one of his patients claimed his child had been conceived a day following the operation. His wife had arrived at the hospital quite concerned about her husband's recovery. She obviously found out about it very quickly!

Apart from this athletic performance in bed, one patient played tennis within 10 days and another skied 11 days after the operation. How soon patients return to activity strictly depends on their own level of pain tolerance. This is because the surgical technique, along with the use of fine steel sutures, guarantees the hernia will not give way.

It was shocking to hear that in other hospitals it's not rare for patients to have the main hernia repaired and return home with one that was neither discovered or repaired. It's hardly what one would expect to happen.

But during a hernia repair at Shouldice, 13 percent of patients are found to have another hernia that was not suspected prior to surgery. These hernias are found because Shouldice surgeons do a layer-by-layer anatomical dissection searching for more than one hernia. These defects are repaired at the same time.

The surgeon explained that these hernias are missed in other hospitals because doctors fail to explore the entire anatomy during surgery. They worry they may damage the spermatic cord which can lead to injury of the testes and legal action. It's another example of how fear of legal action results in a less than perfect procedure.

One of my professors at Harvard gave me sage advice, "To be a success in surgery you have to learn to do one operation well." He was an expert in thyroid surgery. For this reason patients come to Shouldice Hospital from around the world. To be sure, the process is an assembly-line to repair hernias. But wow, what an assembly line!

But is it necessary to repair all hernias? It has always been believed that failing to return the bowel to its normal position inside the abdomen is fraught with danger. Surgeons worried that the bowel would become trapped in the hernia causing intestinal obstruction in which the bowel would become gangrenous and death would occur without emergency surgery. Or that a small hernia would become larger making surgical repair more difficult.

Now a large study has been published in the *Journal of the American Medical Association* that states some hernias are best left alone.

To prove this point five U.S. medical centers followed 700 men with hernias that were causing no or minimal discomfort. Half of the men were selected for a hernia repair. The other 50 percent were told to monitor their symptoms and report back at regular checkups.

To their surprise surgeons discovered that in the hospital group, the most feared complication—intestinal obstruction—occurred in less than one percent of patients per year. This is much better than the odds at Las Vegas. Moreover, any discomfort that was initially present did not increase over a two year period in the majority of cases. Just 25 percent of the "watchful waiting group" asked for surgery due to increased pain. But this delay had no effect on the complication rate such as infection, length of operation or recurrence of hernia.

But what about the other half who were chosen to have the hernia repaired? About 20 percent developed complications after the surgery, such as infection and difficulty passing urine, and three had life-threatening problems. Other studies show that even after a successful hernia repair about five percent of patients continue to have pain. Surgical procedures do not always provide a free lunch.

The Shouldice clinic believes surgeons must get rid of the idea that all hernias must be repaired. This applies particularly to the elderly if they are without discomfort. But age is not a factor as long as the patient is free of cardiovascular disease and other problems that increase the risk. The oldest patients at Shouldice who had a hernia repair was 99!

So we've all heard the phrase, "If it's not broke, don't fix it." Now we can add another equally sound surgical dictum, "If it's only partially broken think twice before you decide to fix it."

This principle also applies to other surgery. For instance, for years parents have been told it was God's will that their children's tonsils should be removed. I'm sure mine were removed at a young age for no good reason. Now we know that this is often needless surgery.

Today CT scans and MRI's often detect gallstones during the diagnosis of other conditions. Or they are discovered unexpectedly during an autopsy. In the past their presence was considered justification for removal. Now we know this is often needless surgery unless the stones are causing symptoms. As I have said before, these gallstones are better left to the crematorium.

I noticed while in training at The Harvard Medical School that I had a tiny hernia. Later I life I developed a slightly larger one on the other side. Neither have caused me any trouble, but I've often wondered if I should have these hernias repaired.

But trying to get a perfect body, particularly when a less than perfect one isn't causing trouble, can result in unintended consequences. As a medical journalist, watching hernia surgery at Shouldice I learned that only a fool would ask for one when it's not causing trouble.

Pitfalls of Surgery

How to Survive a Hospital Stay

Luckily, I've only been admitted to hospital for surgery on two occasions. But when it happened I had serious concerns. The big one was, will I develop a complication during my hospital stay that I didn't have on arrival? So what did I do to prevent this from occurring?

First, I chose my surgeon like porcupines make love, very, very carefully. This choice can have a major impact on outcome. I realize the best of surgeons can encounter a problem that is largely an "Act of God". But chances are slim that an unforeseen problem will occur with a first class technical surgeon. So the surgery is the least of my worries.

I know some of you are saying, "Yes, but you have the inside track and know who to entrust your life to." You're right. Being a surgeon helps, but here's a tip for you. If you're lucky enough to know a scrub nurse, one that assists at surgery, he or she will be able to direct you to the right hands.

Some patients make the mistake of letting emotions determine their hospital choice. They want a particular hospital so friends and family can visit them daily after the operation. Family is important, but not as vital as travelling a few hours to a hospital and surgeon better qualified to do the operation. This emotional decision increases the risk of complications. Remember, the more complicated the surgery, such as brain aneurysm or esophageal malignancy, or removal of a blockage in the carotid artery, the more you need a surgeon who is doing a number of these operations every year. It's the old saying, "practice makes perfect".

My second worry, one that should concern everyone, is the risk of hospital infection. Studies show that in North America what's called "central line infections" are a primary concern. Central line infections are those that occur when patients are receiving antibiotics, medication or nutrition by intravenous needle. This causes up to 30 percent of the 100,000 deaths from infection every year.

Another frequent cause of hospital infection is the use of urinary catheters following surgery. The longer a catheter remains in place, the greater the risk of infection. So always ask the surgeon if the catheter can be removed. Similarly, if you're taking antibiotics, ask when they can be discontinued. The longer you take them the greater risk of complications.

Remain alert to keep needless errors from happening. You obviously can't prevent a sponge or instrument being left in the abdomen. But you can prevent the surgeon from performing the wrong operation. It's prudent, if you're scheduled for a hernia operation, to have the surgeon write his initials on the surgical site. The more caution the better as in rare cases surgeons have operated on the wrong patient or performed the wrong operation!

What's more common are errors of medication. It's no wonder that this happens with so many North Americans taking so many prescription drugs. Numerous traps set the stage for this to happen. Nursing is a tiring job and fatigue can play a role in their service. It's also a dangerous time when the nursing shift changes. A lack of communication has often resulted in a patient receiving the wrong drug or the wrong dose.

How can this error be decreased? According to the health publication, *Consumer Reports on Health*, when nurses were asked this question 87 percent answered, "It would help if patients would bring their list of drugs with them."

Remember, just because you are not a doctor, doesn't mean you lack common sense. Dr. Peter Pronovost, Director of Critical Care at Johns Hopkins School of Medicine provides sage advice. He says, "Question, question, question until things are explained to you in a way you can understand."

Following surgery, get moving as soon a possible. Ships tied up too long develop barnacles. Humans develop clots in their legs that may result in pulmonary embolism and death.

Of course, the best way to prevent surgical complication in hospital is to be sure the operation is needed. Every year thousands of operations are performed for questionable reasons

The main message in getting to 90+ is to keep your mind alert to possible errors during a hospital stay.

Pitfalls of Surgery
Getting Older is Invariably Fatal, Prostate Cancer Only Sometimes

So far prostate cancer has not played any role in my getting to 90+. But having said this, 20 years ago I had to make a decision whether I should or should not have a PSA test. It had become standard practice for doctors to order this test as it made sense to detect early prostate cancer and receive prompt treatment.

But at that time I remembered an old saying, "It's not the things you don't know that gets you into trouble, it's the things you know for sure that ain't so". I was convinced doctors were too sure the new PSA test was worthwhile and harmless. Being skeptical and declining the test probably helped me to get to 90+ without the complications associated with PSA.

This was one time when I rolled the dice and played a little Russian Roulette. This is not an approach I normally use when evaluating medical treatment. I've always had regular colonoscopies as I'm not going to take a chance with this malignancy. But prostate cancer is unusual. It does not play by the rules that apply to other malignancies. Besides, as a medical journalist I was receiving complaints from readers of the unintended consequences of radical prostate surgery such as incontinence and impotence.

I was not alone in making this decision. Years later Richard Albin, the discoverer of the PSA test, publicly stated that he wished he had never developed it. It had resulted in a public health disaster. He admitted the test was imperfect, resulting in too early warnings of malignancy for which treatment was not required. Albin said he himself had never taken a PSA test. Neither have I.

Years later, looking back on my decision, it could have been the wrong one. I might have died from prostate cancer and never reached 90+. But even if the PSA test was abnormal I wasn't sure I wanted to be treated at 70 years of age. Many prostate cancers are slow growing and treatment is often associated with impotence and urinary incontinence. Now, 20 years later, one still needs the Wisdom of Solomon to know who should be treated and who should simply be followed without treatment. This, of course, goes against the basic concept that all cancers should be diagnosed early and promptly treated. But this is no ordinary case. This malignancy can be a pussy cat or a raging tiger.

As I'm about to publish this book, a federal panel of doctors, setting guidelines for cancer screening, has made a headline announcement. They are urging doctors to stop using the PSA test. The panel concluded that the benefit risk–ratio showed that too many patients were being harmed by over-treating early cancers that might never cause death nor symptoms. The panel made its decision in part based on a study conducted in seven countries. In this study only 13 lives were saved for every 10,000 men screened. In effect, 10,000 men would suffer from unintended consequences to save 13 lives. But this report is already being questioned by others who believe the PSA test saves lives. The debate will go on.

In the meantime the following points will show the difficulties doctors face in advising patients on the best treatment.

One

Benjamin Disraeli, Queen Victoria's Prime Minister, once remarked "There are three kinds of lies: lies, damned lies and statistics." Disraeli, if he had been a doctor, could have been referring to the PSA test for prostate cancer. For instance, the *New England Journal of Medicine* just reported a European study that showed that this blood test cut the death rate of this disease by 20 percent. But this impressive figure refers to a relative reduction in deaths.

There's another way to look at the reduction in the number of deaths. 162,000 men were followed for 10 years. Of those given the PSA test, 261 died, compared to 363 deaths of those who received routine care. A difference of 102 deaths out of 162,000 men isn't as impressive.

Another statistic helps patients decide about the value of the PSA test. 1,410 men have to be screened by the PSA test, and an additional 48 men treated, to prevent one prostate cancer death. This means that a massive screening program would have only a modest effect on mortality and some men would get treatment and complications they didn't need.

So statistics can be misleading, or as another wise sage said, "Statistics can be used as drunken men use lamp-posts, for support rather than for illumination."

Two

How many angels can dance on the head of a pin? I don't know the answer to this question. Nor do I, or others, know what is the best treatment for prostate cancer. A young man who is believed to have a rapidly growing malignancy may be advised that a radical prostatectomy is the best chance for survival. For others, external radiation, implanting radium seeds in the prostate gland, or freezing the prostate by cryosurgery may be better options. But at the moment there's no one ultimate treatment that is the best for everyone.

Three

The late Dr. Willett Whitmore, a world authority on prostate cancer at Memorial Hospital in New York City, remarked, "The survival rate has little to do with treatment. Rather it's related to the biological nature of the cancer". In other words, how malignant is the cancer? So pathologists try to grade cancers on how fast they grow. But it's still an inexact science. This presents the great dilemma, how to treat or not to treat prostate cancer?

Four

Hippocrates, the Father of medicine, always stressed when treating the patient, "First, do no harm". This is a huge problem facing doctors who treat patients with prostate cancer.

Five

Suppose you're around 70 years of age and are diagnosed with prostate cancer. It's sometimes better to live with the devil you know than the one you've never met. The devil you know may be a slow growing malignancy and not destined to end your life for many years. In the meantime there's a good chance you will die of something else. By age 70 autopsies show that about 50 percent of males have microscopic cancer cells in their prostate gland. So remember what a world famous urologist once remarked, "Growing older is invariably fatal, cancer of the prostate only sometimes."

Six

The devil you don't know may be a horrible complication resulting from treatment such as impotence or urinary incontinence. Radical prostatectomy is the most frequent cause. Studies show that urinary incontinence is often under-reported, because the person who wets his pants is much more aware of and embarrassed by the annoyance than the surgeon who operated. Many patients who have contacted me over the years mention how difficult it is to live with this problem and would have refused the surgery if they had known of this possible complication. Fortunately surgical techniques have improved which have decreased these complications. For instance, some radical prostatectomies are now being done by robotic surgery.

Seven

Another wise sage said, "If you're not confused about prostate cancer, you don't know what's going on." So my advice is to try as much as possible to be informed about this disease before submitting to treatment. Like Benjamin Disraeli, cast a wary eye at statistics. One of Harvard's most distinguished professors often stated that "If something has to be proven by statistics, it's usually wrong." I say "Amen" to that.

But remember I'm not your doctor and your decision about the PSA test must be made in consultation with your own doctor.

Pitfalls of Surgery

Does Frequent Sex Decrease the Risk of Prostate Cancer?

Hmmm… Why wasn't this study done 70 years ago when I was young with an abundance of testosterone? This was my first reaction to a report in the journal, *Cancer Epidemiology*. But for the Don Juan's of this world, this news is better late than never. I'm sure they will be ecstatic that frequent sex can decrease the risk of prostate cancer. But what will your bride-to-be say?

Marie-Elise Parent is Associate Professor of Epidemiology at the University of Montreal. I have not met her but she's been affectionately called, for appropriate reasons, "Madame Prostate". She has my congratulations for this unique finding.

So what's the good news for Romeos? The Montreal study questioned 3,208 men between 2005 and 2009 on their various lifestyle factors, particularly their frequency of sex. Of this group 1,590 were diagnosed with prostate malignancy. The rest served as the control group.

The study revealed that men who had sex with more than 20 women had 28 percent less risk of developing prostate cancer. But there was more good news. They were also less likely to have a rapid growing form of this disease.

Parent, however, cautioned that this research did not mean men should try to beat the four minute mile getting to the bedroom. Or, that it meant a weekend of unparalleled sex with 20 women. Rather, the amour should be with 20 or more women spaced over a lifetime.

Hmmm… This clarification does have some down-to-earth side-effects and I wonder if Madame Prostate has considered them? For instance, I can imagine the reaction if you said to your bride-to-be, "Darling, this ring means till death do us part. But recent research shows that I'm more likely to die of prostate cancer if I don't have sexual relations with 20 or more women during our marriage. I hope you understand that I still love you and it's not something I want to do. But I'm sure you will agree to this affair in the interest of my health and life."

Maybe readers could pass along to me what the blushing bride-to-be would say!

But the study wasn't all good news. For instance, men who slept with men and who had 20 male partners, had twice the risk of developing prostate cancer than men who never slept with a man. Even worse, their risk of getting a quickly growing prostate malignancy was five times greater.

What about male virgins who had never had sex? They were twice as likely to develop prostate cancer.

The question, apart from the marital disruption this affair would cause, is why romping with 20 or more women would decrease the risk of this often fatal malignancy.

Marie-Elise Parent doesn't know the answer. But she speculates that the frequency of sex with a variety of women increases the sex drive. And increased sex means that during orgasm the concentration of carcinogens is reduced in the prostate gland.

The same theory has been proposed for the prevention of colon cancer. In effect, normal bowel movements decrease the time carcinogens have contact with the wall of the colon and therefore also decrease risk of this disease. But many question this theory and I'm sure many will also question Parent's research.

However, a Harvard study also showed that men who had sex

21 times a month had a 33 percent less risk of prostate cancer than men who had sex 4 to 7 times a month.

Parent says more research on this matter is required. 70 years ago I would have applauded her decision and sacrificed my moral standards in the interest of science to participate in this project. But alas, for those of my age, all we can do is cry in our beer that it is too late to volunteer in this continuing research.

This year 250,000 North American males will be diagnosed with prostate cancer. But since many have a slow growing form of the disease, only 30,000 will die from it. As a world authority aptly remarked, "getting older is invariably fatal, cancer of the prostate only sometimes."

Pitfalls of Depression

Burnout 101 for Caregivers

Here's a possible Trivial Pursuit question, "What's the fastest growing unpaid profession in North America?" I admit I wouldn't have known the answer. But, according to the "Family Caregiver Alliance", more than 65.7 million Americans, that's 29 percent of the population, provide care to a family member, loved one or friend who is ill, disabled or aged. But when does such labour of love trigger burnout anger in the caregiver?

A report from Johns Hopkins University states, "The average unpaid, or informal, caregiver is a 46 year old female with a full or part-time job who spends about 20 hours a week catering for her mother. But for those caring for a loved one older than 65 the average age is 63. Unfortunately, one-third of these caregivers are also in poor health.

Another study carried out in Sweden revealed the shocking news that 18 percent of people older than 75 were involved in the care of others! For these elderly caregivers this isn't what they expected to be doing in their golden years! I'm sure while they're carrying out these arduous daily tasks they must share the thought of the German philosopher Nietzsche who remarked, "There is no greater misery than to remember happier times."

The problem with an aging population is that they suffer from a variety of problems. For instance, a Gallup survey revealed that

15 million North Americans are caring for someone incapacitated by some form of dementia, such as Alzheimer's disease. Millions of others are helping family members suffering from cancer, stroke, multiple sclerosis, Parkinson's disease, or incapacitated by severe unrelenting arthritic pain.

Sooner or later the demands of time and energy made on some caregivers triggers a reaction, similar to the last straw that finally breaks the camel's back. This crisis occurs when they have neglected their own health for too long.

Caring for others is also a dangerous job. For example, in one study caregivers, aged 66 and over, had a 63 percent higher mortality rate than non-caregivers of the same age.

The physical task facing caregivers can be overwhelming. But according to experts it's the mental toll that is more likely to bring caregivers to their knees. They suffer from loneliness, anxiety, fear of the future, depression and at times anger at the person they're caring for. It's small wonder that they require more anti-depressants and anti-anxiety drugs than the general population.

So how can caregivers cope with physical and mental stress day after day? First, it's vital that they don't put their own health at the bottom of the list. This is a sure formula for Burnout 101. Family members must keep a wary eye on the caregiver and realize there's a crisis in the making if they notice her or him reaching for alcohol, having difficulty concentrating, suffering from insomnia or thoughts of suicide. This is a time when other family members must share the burden.

Caregivers who remain silent and uncomplaining are quicker to suffer burnout. It's important for them to "let it out" with a family member, friend, clergy or a counselor. It's also prudent for them to get some form of exercise daily. And to find time during the day for something they enjoy, whether it be reading a book or watching a movie.

Remember that many of the diseases that afflict the elderly have major organizations to provide information on how to handle difficult situations. They also provide support groups in your area.

Caregivers must be ready for emergencies. This means trying to plan ahead for the dangers that could occur in the community. For example, you may live in an area that is prone to sudden snowstorms. What will happen at subzero temperatures if electrical power shuts down for days?

Others who reside in tornado regions need to plan an escape route and how to handle someone in a wheelchair. Moreover, even with a plan of action, you won't get far if the car hasn't an ample supply of gas.

Care giving involves so much work and stress it's no wonder the handler suffers Burnout 101. The bad news is this problem is going to get worse with an aging population.

So far I've been lucky that I, or family members, have not had to face this added stress, another lucky factor that may have added to my longevity.

Pitfalls of Depression

We're Crazy, Not the South Americans

Have you ever had the desire to say, "The hell with it. I'm tired and I don't give a tinker's damn what the boss thinks. I'm closing the door and taking a nap." In our North American society what we want to do (and can do) without getting fired are two different things. But is it time for employers to agree that South Americans are not crazy for shutting their doors and having an afternoon siesta?

Dr. Scott Campbell, a sleep expert at Weill Medical College, in White Plains N.Y., says that "napping is a healthy habit if your schedule permits it. I don't see why you would try to overcome what your body is trying to tell you." I'd agree, but it's safer if the boss is on holiday.

It's the old story that if you don't use it, you lose it. In this case, if you don't snooze, you lose. Besides, there's scientific evidence that napping has benefits. As one wise sage wrote, "No day is so bad it can't be fixed with a nap."

Sleep experts say that our internal clock is programmed to make us sleep twice every 24 hours. The first need for slumber occurs between midnight and 7 a.m. Then the eyelids start to fall again between 1 p.m. and 3 p.m. This biological readiness to sleep in the mid-afternoon also coincides with a slight drop in body temperature. Moreover, this decrease in body temperature occurs whether we eat or not, and even in those who are well rested.

The majority of studies show that even a nap of 15 minutes can increase mental and physical performance. In addition, according to the National Sleep Foundation, short naps boost mood for the remainder of the afternoon which every depressed person needs. This is true regardless of age.

Dr. Campbell reports that a study of 32 men and women between the ages of 55 to 85 found that older people scored higher on tests of cognitive ability and reaction time after napping.

Campbell adds that it's a myth that an afternoon nap interferes with nighttime sleep. It may take a few more minutes to fall asleep at night after napping, but people sleep just as long and deeply as on no nap days. Moreover, their actual sleep time increased by one hour on napping days.

North Americans and employers should realize that napping is a part of our lives right from birth. Moreover, if it's good for healthy toddlers surely a short siesta is even more urgent for those of us with gray hair.

Napping may also be part of an evolutionary, geographical mechanism that evolved in certain cultures, particularly those close to the equator. I'm sure that in South America it didn't take too long for our evolutionary genes to conclude it's prudent to get out of the blistering noonday sun. As Joseph Conrad wrote, "Only mad dogs and Englishmen go out in the noonday sun."

Suppose you're one of the lucky ones who can afford to take a nap without getting fired. Sliding under the desk is not a good idea. Rather, choose a peaceful spot, dim the lights and draw the drapes. Set the alarm if you're concerned about oversleeping. And don't nap longer than 20 to 25 minutes. You may enter a deep sleep after 30 minutes making it more difficult to get back to functioning well. As in most things moderation in napping is the key.

If you can't nap and need energy, avoid sugary treats that just provide a short temporary lift. Rather, select protein and complex carbohydrates such as cheese and whole-wheat crackers. And go easy on caffeinated drinks that can result in dependency.

I was delighted to learn of this research. I'm an early morning writer usually at my computer by 6:00 a.m.. But as sure as night follows day, after lunch I start to yawn at every other word. Then my eyelids start to close and I know it's fruitless to continue. But after a short nap I'm hopefully writing something intelligent. That of course may be a debatable point!

I admit it would be easier selling ice to Eskimos than selling an afternoon nap to employers. But since they're always preaching the need for increased productivity they might find a little nap improves their bottom line.

Pitfalls of Depression
The Dog is Not For Sale

Why did I carry dog biscuits to work on my daily walking commute a few years ago? I admit they're healthier than the occasional hamburger I had for lunch! But the biscuits were for a magnificent German Shepherd dog. He was always with his master, one of the many homeless people begging for money on the streets of Toronto. But why the dog, when his master is unable to feed himself?

Several studies attest to the healing power of pets. A 45 year old quadriplegic who used a mouth stick to operate a computer often dropped it. The problem was solved by a Capuchin monkey who retrieved the stick for her. It also brought her magazines, opened refrigerator doors, put cassettes in the player, and while perched on the arm of a wheelchair, combed her hair. And she was never alone.

Another quadriplegic checked into a Boston hotel. But it was his dog, a black Labrador Retriever, who put his paw on the desk and accepted the room key in his mouth. He also wore a light backpack to carry personal items, pushed elevator buttons and operated light switches.

Are you worried about having a tooth extracted? If so, go to a dentist who has an aquarium. Researchers found that looking at fish in an aquarium prior to removal of a tooth was more effective than hypnosis in calming patient's fears.

In another study, people with normal and high blood pressure were asked to sit in a chair quietly for 20 minutes to stabilize their pressure. Later as they watched fish in an aquarium the blood pressure of those with normal pressures and hypertension dropped to lower levels. This method was as effective in treating hypertension as meditation and biofeedback.

Many studies show that animals have healing power. And it can be lifesaving.

The University of Maryland evaluated the importance of pet ownership in patients with severe coronary artery disease compared to having friends, belonging to a church, social activities and living in friendly neighbourhoods. The results after one year were shocking. Only three of 53 patients with pets died compared to 11 out of 39 patients without pets.

Pet therapy helps to keep healthy people above the ground. The need for people to get off the couch and walk the dog helps to shed pounds.

Dog ownership also provides opportunities for people to make friends. An English study showed that people in neighbourhoods where residents were wary of one another feel safer when a stranger is with a dog. And if you want others to love you, have your picture taken with a dog. Politicians have long known of this benefit.

Researchers have also studied the effects of pet therapy on prisoners. Initially small caged animals such as birds, rabbits and hamsters were introduced to some criminals. During the next year the level of prison violence decreased and suicide attempts ceased entirely. The interaction with animals appeared to establish trust and increased communication among inmates. And dogs never ask what crime they committed.

Pets can also improve people's social lives. One of my patients who had lost her husband told me each year of her loneliness and boredom. But one year she returned in good spirits. While exercising with her dog in a park she met a man who was also walking his dog. Now they were happily married. Even the dogs were happier!

I admit that after many months I had fallen for the German Shepherd on the corner, and like to think he liked me too. Perhaps I was being naïve. He may have liked me just for the biscuits. But there's no doubt he loved his master unconditionally, without any thought of his race, economic circumstances, or physical appearance.

But how much did his master love him? He was well fed even without the biscuits. And in the bitter cold he always had his coat on. But when I passed him, I always wondered if a man asking for money would sell his dog. One day I asked him.

I was pleased to hear his handsome German Shepherd was not for sale. "Not at any price." Money could never replace the comfort that dog gave his master day after day.

Pitfalls of Depression

This Haircut Will Cost Me a Lot of Money

"Would you like a free massage after your haircut, doctor?" the owner of Elizabeth Milan's salon in Toronto's Royal York Hotel asked me. It had been a long day seeing patients and maybe I looked a trifle haggard. But whatever the reason, being of Scottish heritage, the 'free' part appealed to me. So I said, "Why not?"

Massage as therapy has stood the test of time. It's been used by the Chinese, Greeks, Roman and Indian civilizations. During a trip to Egypt last year I saw numerous paintings of people practicing massage in the tombs of Kings and Queens. And Julius Caesar was apparently given daily massage to treat neuralgia.

Many people tend to look on massage as a luxury found only in upscale health clubs. But massage is a great tool, a combination of art and science. It can have a major impact in treating tension, insomnia, headache, hypertension, arthritis, acute and chronic pain and can promote healing in a variety of conditions.

How does it work? Research shows the enormous benefit of hands-on therapy. It fosters a positive emotional reaction to physical touch designed to ease whatever ails you. That's why the massage therapist has so much more to offer psychologically and physically than a doctor who simply hands out prescriptions across a desk.

But there's more to massage than the touch of well-trained

hands. Massage, by manipulating tissues, muscles and tendons decreases stress hormones, enhances the production of endorphins, the body's natural painkillers, and by improving circulation eases muscle spasm and joint stiffness. Besides all this, it makes you feel good, and how do you weigh that benefit?

A report from The Mayo Clinic claims that massage has reduced anxiety in depressed children. This finding should be sent to every school in this country that believes hyperactive children are best treated by sedating them with drugs.

Years ago when I was hyperactive in school I was sedated by a good whack on my backside. I don't believe this has caused me psychological harm. But in retrospect I would have preferred to be sedated by a relaxing massage.

The Mayo Clinic adds that studies show massage results in reduced pain in those suffering from fibromyalgia, recent surgery, and back pain. And we all know its benefits in sport injuries.

It's interesting that massage has produced weight gain in premature infants and decreased the number of days they were required to stay in hospital. Other children with diabetes who received daily massage were more likely to stick to their medication and diet.

In other studies, cancer patients undergoing treatment also reported less anxiety and pain if they had regularly scheduled massage sessions.

I can't confirm this fact, but I'd bet my last dollar that those with terminal illness would find their days less painful and depressing if massage were part of their treatment.

How did I fare after my treatment? I felt relaxed and ready to take on the world. But I had a problem. There was no suggestion that the next session would be free. That triggered considerable tension. Unfortunately I'll have to pay to find out how much anxiety and insomnia it will cause me.

But I'm sure that if one massage provides so much help, frequent massages would do even more. So in the end this free massage is going to cost me a lot of money. Hopefully I can get my psyche to accept massage, not as an expense item, rather an investment in relaxation and good health in an increasingly tense world where so many problems are related to stress.

Massage is also non-invasive, without any of the side effects of drug therapy. It's therefore a great way to help decrease the frightening epidemic of "pillitis" in this country. If doctors wrote more prescriptions for massage there would be fewer written for antidepressant drugs.

This is why for years I've avoided both non-prescription and prescription medication unless there's good reason for taking them. They all have to be metabolized by the liver and excreted by the kidneys. Overworking and abusing these organs is never a good idea. You have a greater chance of reaching 90+ the more often you say "no thanks" to the doctor prescribing an unnecessary drug.

Napoleon Bonaparte, hardly a role model for saving lives, nevertheless had the right idea about pills when he remarked, "Take one dose of medicine once, and in all probability you will be obliged to take an additional hundred thereafter". "Amen" to that.

Pitfalls of Depression

10 Ways I've Handled Stress for 90+ Years

Voltaire was right when he wrote, "Most people live lives of quiet desperation." As we enter another year, desperation seems to be getting worse. Escalating violence in the Middle East, journalists being beheaded, concern about our economy, worry, etc, etc. So here are some sound ways to help decrease tension in 2015.

One

Massage cures more stress and sore muscles than a cartload of pills. This message has not been lost on an industry where anything to help the bottom-line becomes top priority. Some companies are now using massage as a form of stress management to decrease fatigue, headache and back strain in their employees. This results in greater employee retention and job satisfaction. Remember that athletes and boxers don't get rub-downs just for show business. Muscle activity burns glycogen which in turn produces lactic and carbonic acid. Massage helps to remove these toxic products of metabolism.

Two

Joseph Stalin, one of the worst despots of all time, at least gave good advice when he remarked, "One has to live with the devil until you reach the end of the bridge." You have to learn to separate the possible from the impossible. Every week in my office I used to see emotional problems that a trainload of psychiatrists couldn't cure. If you have an idiotic boss who should never have been promoted, there's usually no way to tell him or her to go to hell unless you win the lottery. And if your partner has run off with your best friend only time will heal the psychological trauma. So play for time rather than trying to solve an unsolvable problem.

Three
A study at The Harvard Medical School showed that students who meditated for 15 minutes a day or played solitaire, knitted, read a book or engaged in aerobic exercise inoculated themselves against modern day anxieties more than students who failed to take the time for distraction.

Four
Laughter is a great way to decrease stress. Years ago Norman Cousins, editor of *The Saturday Review*, was stricken with a crippling illness that involved his joints. He decided to treat himself with laughter and day after day watched humourous movies. Eventually, his health was restored and for years after he taught the value of laughter at The University of California Medical School. It's been aptly said that if it were not for laughs we might be sicker than we are. And no one to my knowledge has ever died from laughter.

Five
Remember that life without stress is death. The late Hans Selye, President of The International Institute of Stress, cautioned patients that since tension cannot be totally escaped, they should attempt to keep it within normal limits. And to realize when the

threshold has been passed, to seek medical help if they experience palpitations, headaches and insomnia. His message was to practice "pace, not race."

Six

Learn to live with less. It's conceivable that life would still go on without the latest electronic gadget. Saving for a rainy day saves a lot of stress.

Seven

Don't forget the psychological and physiological benefits of sex. It's one of the best tranquillizers available. After all, who doesn't sleep like a baby after sex? And since we all worry about getting older here's more good news. Dr. David Weeks, a neuropsychologist at Scotland's Royal Edinburgh Hospital studied 3,500 people ranging in age from 18 to 102. He concluded that frequent sex slows the aging process! Even if he's wrong what do you have to lose?

Eight

Try to believe the bottle is half full, not half empty. And stop "catastrophizing and awfulizing."

Nine

Be realistic about expectations, thereby decreasing the disappointment factor.

Ten

Tense patients look surprised when I say to them, "Take a train ride. It's a great way to relax." This past Christmas, rather than face the turmoil of airports, my wife and I boarded Via Rail for Montreal and savoured the delights of Old Montreal. Another short Via Rail trip took us to historic Chateau Frontenac hotel in Quebec City. We walked the ramparts of the citadel, enjoyed the ambiance of this great city and practiced what I preach, that wine increases good cholesterol. Another time we rode the rails across Canada. It provides ample time to read books and relax. Try it. You might like it. And at 90+ it's stress free.

Pitfalls of Depression

How I Escaped Depression

"How have you been able to avoid being depressed?" several friends have asked me. They know that over the years as a medical journalist I've had some dicey moments with opposition. So the question is a good one with no single answer. But I've always remembered and admired Harry Truman, former President of the U.S.. Truman shot from the hip and called a spade a spade. When discussing what it was like being President, he accepted that criticism was part of the job. He remarked, "If you can't stand the heat, get out of the kitchen!" He once added, when talking to the Press Club in Washington, "if you need a good friend, go buy a dog."

I believe I escaped depression because I also knew criticism was part of the job of a syndicated medical journalist. Particularly, as my genetic makeup prohibits my sitting on-the-fence when writing about controversial socio-medical issues. I believe these are the very issues that should be discussed, and vital to our society.

This means that along the way I've faced some difficult times. I discovered you get scars on your back even when the general population agrees with your opinion. For instance, when I decided to try to legalize heroin in Canada to ease the agony of terminal cancer patients, I thought humanitarian organizations would applaud this move. Why? Because it had been used to treat terminal cancer patients in England for over 90 years. But

I was immediately damned by the Canadian Cancer Society, the RCMP, hospital pharmacists, and received no help from the medical establishment.

The four-year battle is documented in my book *"You're Going To Do What?"* Suffice to say, I spent time researching this issue in England and Scotland. It revealed that heroin was not only being used to help cancer patients both young and old, but also women in difficult childbirth, burn patients and accident victims. It was administered quickly to those in emergency units suffering from coronary attack. Heroin was finally legalized in Canada for terminal cancer patients in February 1984. But due to bureaucratic red tape the use of heroin was difficult to prescribe and the company importing heroin ceased to do so.

I did not descend into a depressive funk, but I was annoyed that so much time and effort had been expended uselessly to relieve pain and suffering. I won't tell you what I hope happens to those who were responsible for this tragedy. It should never have happened.

Over the years some controversial columns triggered threats to my life. Rather than face depression, my response tended to grow more positive. I decided to continue provoking rational thought rather than quit the heat of the kitchen.

As I look back on my life it became a challenge to fight for common sense, an uncommon commodity. As I wrote in the Globe and Mail years ago, "The problems in society are being committed by so-called intelligent people who are largely fools." I'm convinced that keeping busy and focussed on today's social problems leaves little time for depression. Or if it's been a bad day and I'm annoyed at asinine criticism, I quickly recover by remembering this sage remark, "Nil Illegitimi Carborundum" which translates, "Don't Let The Bastards Grind You Down."

I do realize, however, that some people face black depression day after day. This is far beyond the range of my expertise. As we have seen so many times some of these patients, who can afford the best of psychiatric care, nevertheless end up taking their own lives. So much to live for, but overwhelmed by depression, they reach the point of desperation with no relief.

As Dante wrote, "There is no greater grief than, in misery, to recall happier times."

Pitfalls of Sexual Behaviour

Want to Be Shot by a Jealous Lover at 95

Can a good sex life increase the chance of getting to 90+? This is a tough question, as I have spent my life as a surgeon, not a sexologist. So although I've written over 2,000 columns, only a few medical ones relate to this topic. But when patients sought advice about sex I always reminded them that sex is only five percent of a marriage, but stressed it is the first five percent. I hoped this remark got the message across that sex was not to be neglected and that sometimes you had to work at it. Good sense should also tell us that a little romp in the bed is of psychological and even physical help.

But you will see in this chapter that the *British Medical Journal* presents scientific evidence that if you want to get to 90 +, sex is one way to help you achieve that goal. In effect, weight lifting or running the four minute mile is not the only way to stay in shape and enjoy longevity.

Some readers may be annoyed at my mentioning the use of cardiac defibrillators in Swiss brothels. Or they may be shocked that I would ever consider ending my 90 + years in the Thorupgaarden nursing home. But I'm a very practical person. Why not a defibrillator in a brothel if it saves lives? And would I elect to be in a sterile Canadian nursing home sitting in a rocking chair compared to having a Saturday evening at Thorupgaarden? I'll let you decide.

So since sex has toppled empires and is a potent force in a good relationship, the best way to obtain my opinion on sex is to read the following columns. Maybe you will even have a little chuckle, which never killed anyone. And realize that my idea of being shot by a jealous lover is not a bad way to go!

Pitfalls of Sexual Behaviour
Eight Good Reasons to Make Love

Are you fed up reading about war, our failing health care system and crooked CEOs? If so, let's discuss a more pleasant topic, the way to ensure a long and healthy life. Some are convinced that jogging, a variety of diets or a daily glass of red wine is the answer. But what about sex? The fact is that making love is downright good for you. Here are eight reasons why you should put more amore into your life.

It's Good Exercise
Since making love involves some interesting acrobatics, having sex three times a week burns about 7,500 calories in a year. This is the equivalent of jogging 75 miles! And vigorous sex consumes up to 200 calories each time. At three times a week this activity consumes 31,000 calories a year, the same as 300 miles of jogging. Given this choice why would anyone want to jog? After all, making love is usually a pleasant affair. But have you ever seen a jogger smiling? They look like they're about to take their last breath.

Decreases the Risk of Dying
It's been said that the French have sex lives, the English have hot water bottles! But what about the Irish? Researchers at Queens

University in Belfast, Ireland, tracked the mortality of 1,000 middle-aged men over the course of 10 years. They reported in the *British Medical Journal* that men who had the highest frequency of sex enjoyed a death rate 50 percent less than those who were less sexually active. The French, unlike the Irish, don't need a scientific study to reach this conclusion. They call orgasm, "la petite mort." or the little death. But they are quick to add that, a little death now and then can help to postpone the big one! As I examine this research, sex seems a small price to pay for extending one's life!

Reduced Risk of Heart Disease

Another aspect of the study at Queen's University showed that sex improves cardiovascular health. Men who were having sex three or more times a week cut their risk of heart attack in half. Shah Ebrahim, co-author of this study, displayed the British gift of understatement when he remarked, "The relationship between frequency of sexual intercourse and mortality is of considerable public interest." And, I would add, of great personal interest.

Pain Relief

Dr. BeverlyWhipple, Associate Professor at Rutgers University, says sex can help to relieve the pain of arthritis, whiplash and other injuries. During sex, levels of the hormone oxytocin surges to five times its normal level. This in turn releases endorphins, the body's own morphine. So for those who say they have a headache, have sex and the pain may be gone after it.

Prevents Chronic Prostatitis

During orgasm the muscles around the prostate gland contract pushing out prostate fluid which keeps the gland healthy. It's often said "use it or you lose it." But lack of use may also cause chronic prostatitis, an enlargement of the gland associated with annoying chronic pain in the rectal area.

Less Frequent Colds

Wilkes University in Pennsylvania claims that individuals who have sex once or twice a week show 30 percent higher levels of an antibody called immunoglobulin A, which is known to boost the immune system.

Relieves Stress

Today, too many people are reaching for anti-depressants and sleeping pills to treat anxiety and insomnia. But this medication often causes side effects. They forget the remedy may be found in the bedroom. Normal sex is 100 percent natural, without side effects, lessens tension and encourages sleep.

Bonds Couples

I often tell patients that sex is only five percent of a marriage, but the first five percent. For years young couples have been led to believe that having husbands participate in birth in the delivery bonds the marriage. I have always felt (although few agree with me) that this practice is scientific nonsense but it's still going on. The idea was initially started as a marketing device by some U.S hospitals and later this practice spread to Canada. Now, we're seeing these labour room bonded marriages breaking apart. So much for that experiment. A good sex life does more to bond a marriage than witnessing a thousand baby deliveries.

Pitfalls of Sexual Behaviour

Sex After a Heart Attack?

I've always believed that being shot at 95 years of age by a jealous lover is the ideal way to depart this earth. But suppose you survive a coronary attack much earlier in life. How is it going to affect your sex life? Is it time to forget about "amour" and switch to backgammon or hooking rugs? Or, is a little romp in the bed still safe?

Dr. Randal Thomas, Director of the Cardiovascular Health Clinic at The Mayo Clinic says, "A person's life is essentially thrown upside-down following coronary attack. He sees his frailty and how close he came to dying, and it can lead to a lot of psychological issues and need for recuperation."

Another cardiologist, Nieca Goldberg at Lennox Hill Hospital in New York City, says "female patients worry about increased heart rate and sweating during sex after a heart attack." She adds that "sex sidelines many patients after a coronary, especially women, and that they have higher rates of depression."

Goldberg says that some patients simply give up sex after a heart attack and are too embarrassed to talk to their doctor about it.

So you're getting a little frisky and wonder how long you have to wait before having sex. Guidelines issued by The Princeton Consensus Panel stress that sexual activity is too risky during the first two weeks after a heart attack. But that 70 percent of patients are at low risk for a coital heart attack and can resume sexual activity within three to four weeks. The other 30 percent may require further testing before being given the green light.

A study reported in the *Journal of The American Medical Association*, followed 1,774 heart attack patients. It found that for patients at highest risk there was only a 20 in 1,000,000 chance of having a second heart attack during sex. This is certainly better than the odds of winning in Las Vegas. In fact, they claimed that anger was three times more likely than sexual activity to trigger another coronary death.

Another study at the University of Maryland found that even men suffering from chronic heart failure could safely engage in sexual activity.

But what actually happens in the real world? Some coronary patients never say die and have to prove their sexual prowess at the first opportunity. At a recent medical meeting, a speaker reported that one patient in a private room had engaged in sex the day after the heart attack! That must be one for *The Guinness Book of Records*. But it might also be one for the next morning newspaper's obituary page.

For the less adventuresome, sex after a heart attack is a worrying time. Some fear sudden death during or following intercourse. And you can bet that if the person who had the heart attack isn't worried, his or her partner will be anxious. After all, who wants to be responsible for triggering a second coronary and possibly death in the bedroom?

But this should not be a major worry for most people, nor the need to put sex on the back burner. After all, studies show you don't need the same energy as running in a marathon race. Experts say that intercourse expends about as much energy as walking 2 to 3 miles per hour or climbing two flights of stairs. So most people should just consider sex an enjoyable workout.

However, a word of caution. I too have no desire to be responsible for death in the bedroom. Never use sex as a way to enter *The Guinness Book of Records* following heart attack. Moreover, if you're planning a clandestine affair after coronary attack, remember that studies show the stress associated with cheating increases the risk of heart attack. Nelson Rockefeller discovered that fact the hard way.

Finally, if you develop chest pain, an irregular heart rate or excessive shortness of breath during sex, don't push your luck. Stop and see your doctor. That is unless you're lucky enough to have reached 95 years of age. It may be the best way to go.

Pitfalls of Sexual Behaviour
Senior Sex and Saturday Night at Thorupgaarden

One university survey recently revealed that 80 per cent of students thought their parents didn't have any "amour". Talk about child denial! Society in general seems to believe that seniors just pull up the covers and go to sleep. But sex shouldn't go off the radar at age 60, 80 or even in a nursing home. Besides, the Danes have discovered that sex even decreases the cost of medical care. North Americans should take note.

Sure, sexual activity changes as you get older. You may no longer hang from the chandelier while having sex. But for some couples, slowing down and being less acrobatic enhances the experience. Besides, 50 percent of people over 50 are either widowed or divorced and in need of tender-loving-care.

Years ago a song titled, "Saturday night is the loneliest night of the week" was popular. But at Thorupgaarden nursing home in Copenhagen, Denmark, it's not lonely anymore.

I couldn't stop reading about this nursing home. I just wish I had been a fly on the wall when staff were debating its earth-shaking proposal. They decided, in their infinite wisdom, that pornography had a more calming effect on seniors than Prozac. So every Saturday night pornographic videos are available on the home's internal program.

But before my proper readers go into a state of shock, I'd suggest they sit down before hearing of the next decision. If some residents continue to feel lonely and remain depressed after viewing pornographic videos, there's no need to despair. Residents can go the next step and request that a prostitute be allowed to visit. Wow, can you imagine that happening in this country?

But the Danes believe such measures are logical. A spokesperson for the Danish Seniors Lobby Group says pornography is healthier, more economic and easier to use than medication. If you walk into many senior facilities on this continent you will witness seniors half-drugged, depressed and immobile. I believe she has a point.

So how has this unorthodox treatment been accepted by the Danes and residents? Maj-Britt, a department head at Thorupgaarden, says that sexuality is often overlooked in nursing homes. Moreover, there's only been one complaint since the videos program started three years ago. Danish gerontologists (those who specialize in caring for the elderly) also agree with this practice,

What about political reaction? I say kudos to the Danish government. It issued a report confirming that sexuality is an integral part of life for both seniors and disabled people. It agreed with the caregivers.

As many readers know, I believe that alcohol in moderation is a beneficial medicine for many symptoms. And that a pub in every hospital would do more good than a cartload of the pills prescribed for seniors. A wee tipple along with occasional sex might cut down on the mandatory nightly sleeping pill that whacks patients into never-never land.

Of course I'm against child pornography. I'm also convinced that the overall morality of this nation has gone to hell. But I believe we should get over the tendency to label seniors who are interested in sex as "dirty old men" or "dirty old women."

No doubt I have shocked some readers. But at least this column may have kept you from dozing off. Remember, it's the job of a journalist to make people think. Possibly remind them that we should never ask for whom the bell tolls. One day some of us may be sitting in a lonely room looking at four blank walls. No doubt we will be bored as hell and desperate for a little excitement. We might even conclude that the Danes were much more realistic and that a pornographic movie on a Saturday night wasn't such a bad idea.

Since I've never sat on the fence with contentious issues, would I apply for a bed at Thorupgaarden in my dotage? Yes, as it seems to be a lively place on Saturday night. Besides, now at 90+, when my time comes I'd prefer being with a lady-of-the-night and a glass of Chardonnay than falling out of my rocking chair.

Will this ever happen in this country? Hell will freeze over first.

Pitfalls of Sexual Behaviour
Do Men Need the Big "T" for ED?

I would have loved to interview Mae West: singer, playright, vaudevillian and movie sex queen of years ago. She was smart and had a handful of funny quotes in her routine. "Sex is like good bridge" she'd say. "If you don't have a good partner, you'd better have a good hand." Or "sex is emotion in motion." She also loved moralists who went after her steamy, sexual settings by saying, " I believe in censorship. I made a fortune out of it."

Mae West might even have a good cure for males who have lost the "tiger-in-the-tank." The ones who are more irritable, suffer insomnia, have problems at work, lost height, lack energy and lack erections. Then they wonder if testosterone therapy is what's needed to restore their male vigour.

Maybe her sultry voice would cure them when greeted by one of her one-liners, "Is that a gun in your pocket, or are you happy to see me?" But since Mae West is no longer around, what about the use of testosterone?

I first became interested in what's often called "the big T" years ago when I interviewed Dr. Malcolm Carruthers at a Conference on Aging in London, England. Carruthers, a distinguished Harley Street specialist, was one of the early pioneers in testosterone therapy.

During the interview with Carruthers, I met one of his patients who had just received a second testosterone injection. He admitted to me that, following the first injection, he had made love three times in 24 hours!

Needless to say he was a happy camper, and if you want to be shot by a jealous lover at 95 years of age, this is the way to achieve that goal!

But will you reach 95 if you take testosterone? It's been aptly said, "All would be well if there were no buts." The problem is there has always been, and still is a debate as to whether a testosterone boost increases the risk of prostate cancer, stroke or heart attack.

Carruthers has treated over 2,000 men with testosterone. He says, "The myth about testosterone being linked to prostate cancer has been deeply rooted in medical consciousness for over 60 years without this happening."

But what about heart attack?

I also interviewed Dr. Peter Collins, Professor of Cardiology at the Imperial College of Science and Medicine in London, England. He is also a leading expert on testosterone and coronary heart disease.

Collins, like Carruthers, believes that linking testosterone to heart attack is wrong. In fact, he claims mounting evidence shows that normal amounts of testosterone protect against it.

For instance, Collins' research shows that testosterone increases coronary blood flow by as much as 15 to 20 percent. This is why patients suffering from angina (heart pain that increases with exercise) can be helped by testosterone treatment. In addition, testosterone also decreases blood cholesterol and fibrinogen, the small particles that form blood clots.

Dr. Eugene Shippen, a U.S. expert on testosterone pathology, claims that those suffering from erectile dysfunction (ED) are often suffering from low blood testosterone. These men, he claims, are two to three times more likely to suffer a heart attack or stroke.

This evidence supplements the work of Dr. Steven Grover, Professor of Medicine at McGill University, Montreal. He suggests "impotence is the alarm bell for a heart attack."

He adds that, "In approximately 25 percent of cardiovascular patients their first symptom of heart disease is that they drop dead." This is not an encouraging warning and all the more reason to find a sign to indicate an attack is imminent.

Dr. Grover's study compared 4,000 men with and without cardiovascular disease. It showed that men with this problem had a 54 percent chance of having ED than those without cardiovascular disease.

Also not well known is that testosterone helps to fight one of the nation's big killers, diabetes. Type 2 diabetes patients often develop insulin resistance. They possess adequate amounts of insulin, but their cells refuse to accept it. It's like having gas in the car, but the engine won't use it. Testosterone increases the effectiveness of insulin.

So is it testosterone or not? You need the wisdom of Solomon to know who is right. What is thought to be true today may not be so tomorrow.

But one thing appears to be certain. Dr. Carruthers claims he can cure 65 percent of those suffering ED by testosterone therapy alone. The other 35 percent show a 95 percent chance they can be helped by the combination of testosterone along with other erectile dysfunction drugs such as Viagra, Cialis and Levitra.

But if even this fails, there's always Mae West to be seen on YouTube!

Pitfalls of Radiation

Why I've Said "No" to Needless Radiation

For me getting to 90+ has been the result of many things. It's been said that even the street dog has his lucky days. Good luck has kept me away from many diseases over which I have no control. But I did have control over needless radiation. I've avoided it whenever possible.

It's been said that elephants never forget. Neither does radiation. The human body has a natural computer that records every bit of radiation to which it is exposed during a lifetime. Studies show that the greater the amount of radiation received the greater the risk of developing a malignancy.

One of the problems facing both doctors and patients is that an increasing number of tests require radiation. This can result in an earlier diagnosis of cancers and non-malignant problems. But this also means one has to consider the risk-benefit ratio which is often not an easy decision. Most authorities agree that many of the radiation procedures are ordered for questionable reasons. And in the process, although some patients will be helped, a larger number will be exposed to needless radiation.

One of the best examples is the use of radiation in the diagnosis of lung cancer. This malignancy kills more people than prostate, breast and colon cancer combined. Only 15 percent of those diagnosed with lung cancer are alive in five years. So this is good reason for early diagnosis. But when a headline screams, " CT Scans Decrease Lung Cancers Deaths by 20 Percent," it looks like an impressive figure and an irresistible procedure, but it's misleading the public.

One study involved 53,000 current and previous smokers, aged 55 to 74 years. Half of this group received a CT Scan annually, the other half were followed by the standard chest X-rays. Researchers then followed both groups for eight years. During this time 442 smokers died using the standard chest X-rays and 354 who had CT scans. This is not a huge difference. Or as another headline noted "300 CT Scans needed to save one life."

The cost of this study was 250 million dollars. But money is not the only factor when a doctor suggests a CT Scan. One CT Scan results in the same amount of radiation as 500 standard chest X-rays. The question is how many people, knowing this fact, would agree to this number of X-rays? Those patients who were followed for eight years by CT Scans received the level of radiation of 4,000 chest X-rays! So there is a price to pay for earlier diagnosis. But suppose it's a young child who has a CT Scan. Children's organs are more sensitive and a single CT Scan of the stomach is equivalent to 4,000 X-rays! In effect, children are being exposed to levels of radiation that are believed to cause cancer.

There's another problem. CT Scans are much like a microscope. The greater the power of the microscope the more detail can be detected. That's the good news. The bad news is the CT Scan detects small masses. It's sometimes impossible to tell if the mass is a cancer or some other non-malignant problem such as scar tissue. This is called a false positive test which creates a dilemma. The only recourse is to remove the lesion or do a biopsy. This means entering the chest cavity, not a minor procedure. The end result may be good news but it means a large number of patients have a procedure they did not need, and which may result in a surgical complication.

It's been said that if you give a carpenter a hammer he will want to drive in nails. Give doctors new expensive techniques and they will want to use them as sure as the sun will rise tomorrow morning.

This is exactly what has happened. In the U.S. 10 years ago doctors ordered 30 million CT Scans. Last year in 2014 the number had jumped to 80 million. And no one knows how many malignancies will result from this radiation, or from that required for CT angiography to detect coronary artery disease.

So what about the wisdom of a full body CT Scan? One Hawaiian resort markets the procedure for "Peace of Mind" service. Another clinic says it is the "Walmart for CT Scans." This is Marketing 101 at its extreme for people who don't feel well and wonder if they have a life-threatening disease. Or if their nagging pain is due to a malignancy or an impending heart attack? Some clinics in the U.S., in spas or shopping malls, now advertise that it's possible to eliminate all these fears by having a full body scan.

Of course, there is the possibility that this procedure might detect an abdominal aortic aneurysm before it ruptures and kills you. Or it could diagnose blockage of a coronary artery or an unsuspected malignancy. So many would ask, what have you to lose?

A report from the Mayo Clinic stresses that choosing a full body scan requires more thought than deciding on a beauty treatment. Some clinics have substandard equipment which leaves people with a false sense of security. And thinking themselves perfect, may forgo their regular physical examinations. But full body scans are not always perfect. Nor are the radiologists who read them. And we know that about 80 percent of abnormalities found in the scan are of no importance.

General agreement is that full body scans are very questionable and often create more trouble than they solve, not to mention the risk of radiation.

If a doctor suggests a CT Scan, it's prudent to ask if it's really necessary. What could happen if it isn't done? How much radiation will you receive? And if it is necessary, can you have a copy of the report to give to another doctor to avoid another CT Scan. And is it possible to get the same information by either an ultrasound or an MRI which does not expose you to ionizing radiation?

What about dental X-rays? My dentist knows I only want them only when it's very necessary. Even more important, children should be protected from excess radiation.

Dr. Elizabeth Claus of Yale University reports a link between dental X-rays and the development of a brain tumour called a meningioma. She studied patients who had meningiomas and those who did not. She concluded that those who had full mouth X-rays before 10 years of age were 4.9 times more likely to develop a meningioma. And those who had full mouth X-rays later than 10 years of age were three times more prone to this tumour. This should flash a red light for parents.

According to Dr Klaus all children who get braces today also get full mouth X-rays. The question is how many of these children really need braces and has this practice become a fashionable trend? Is the risk worthwhile if it's only for cosmetic reasons?

In the meantime everyone should use common sense about all kinds of radiation. For instance, some experts feel we are living in Alice's Wonderland when we ignore the radiation of cell phones.

The Environmental Health Trusts Newsletter reports this unusual case. A young woman with no predisposing risk of cancer decided to carry her cell phone in her bra. I applaud her for ingenuity and increased security. But unfortunately she developed breast cancer. What shocked doctors was that the pattern of the cancer lined up perfectly with the shape of her cellphone. This does not prove that radiation caused the malignancy. But if I were a woman I would not push my luck. I'd choose another location to carry my cell phone. And children should not be allowed to sleep with a cell phone under their pillow.

I wonder how many people understand that after nuclear tests or after radiation for cancer, that it's possible to pass along radiation to others. During scans to detect thyroid disease, coronary blockage and cancer, doctors use radioactive drugs. Gamma cameras or positron emission tomography (PET) scanners can then detect this energy and use it to produce images on a computer.

Because of this exposure to radiation doctors advise patients to wash their hands well after using the toilet. It's also important to flush the toilet twice to get rid of any radioactive material.

There are varying degrees of radiation. For instance, patients having external radiation should know that beams of radiation focused on a cancer will not spread radiation to other people.

Internal radiation is another matter, particularly when prostate cancers are treated by brachytherapy. During this procedure radioactive pellets, about the size a grain of rice, are injected into prostate tissue. A report from Johns Hopkins says that if low dose pellets are used, patients require a hospital stay. During this time they should have limited contact with family members. Friends should stay for only 15 to 30 minutes and pregnant women should stay away.

But it's another story if doctors implant permanent brachytherapy implants which gradually degrade over time. Radiation experts say patients should not hug family members or others who want to wish them well for a few days following implantation. And for six months they should stay six feet away from children and pregnant women.

Radioactive iodine is also used to treat an overactive thyroid and thyroid malignancy. In this situation, for the first week after treatment, the patient must sleep alone, use separate towels and dishes and wash clothes separately. And following a bone or thyroid scan the body emits radiation for up to three days.

But how often are patients advised that they are radioactive? *The Journal of Nuclear Medicine* reported that a survey of 66 healthcare facilities revealed that often patients had no idea they were emitting radiation.

I have reported for years that everyone should have a radiation card that shows how much radiation was received with each procedure. But it appears hell will freeze over before this happens.

Pitfalls of Exercise
Lions Don't Buy Nike Running Shoes

Have you ever seen lions running? You bet they run when they're hungry and chasing prey. The only other time they exercise is during mating season when they're having sex every 20 minutes! But most of the time they lay around or sleep. Exercise is simply not high on their priority list and they survive well without buying Nike running shoes.

Questioning the value of exercise to humans, however, is like damning Motherhood and apple pie. But every year in my office I see examples of excessive exercise causing needless injury and many aggravating problems.

One of my 60 year old female patients decided it was time to build up muscles. She hired a personal trainer. At each visit she enthusiastically told me how her trainer kept adding extra weights for her leg lifts. I advised her not to push her luck. But the weights kept piling on and on. Finally something snapped. Now she has a partially paralyzed left foot. She should have listened to the old sage who counselled, "Too much of anything can be worse than none at all." And that, at her age, she wasn't meant to be a weight lifter.

Another example of overuse is Olympic athletes. On TV screens they appear to be at the peak of physical form, lean, muscled and full of youth. But they all push themselves to extremes, playing through pain and often undergoing multiple operations due to injuries. Some end up with hips and knees of people twice their age.

Jordan Metzl, of the Sports Medicine Institute for Young Athletes at the Hospital for Special Surgery in New York, says, "We see people 16 years of age with the bones of a 60 to 70 year old person."

Another instance, teenage gymnasts often experience late puberty due to intense exercise and low body fat. But subjecting themselves to this routine before their body is fully developed can lead to lower bone density, osteoporosis and stress fractures.

Marcia Whalen, an osteopathic physician in California, and one of the physicians for the U.S. Women's Olympic Water Polo Team, says, "When you're doing any kind of activity repetitively over and over the way these athletes are doing, it's a set-up for injury." It's also a set-up for the rest of us who overdo it.

Myra Cocker, a researcher at the Stephenson Cardiovascular Centre in Calgary, has been using imaging techniques to study athlete's hearts. It was hoped she and her colleagues would discover why some athletes in superb condition suffer sudden cardiac arrest and die. What they found was equally alarming.

48 Olympic caliber athletes with a median age of 32 years were enlisted in the study. They were involved in swimming, cross country skiing, skating and marathon running. Contrast-enhanced cardiovascular magnetic resonance scans were then done on the athletes. In addition, the same study was carried out on eight others in good health, but who were not involved in a training schedule.

This study showed that 75 percent of the elite athletes had myocardial fibrosis (scarring of the heart's muscle). They also had large ventricles (chambers of the heart). At the moment it's not known what effect this finding will have on longevity. But they believe this scarring will prevent them from ever becoming world champions regardless of how hard they train.

Of course I'm not against moderate exercise when so many today are obese couch potatoes. But I think Abraham Lincoln was right when he said, "The best two doctors are your right and left leg." Walking, a moderate exercise, is still the best one.

So who wins the race in terms of longevity and good health? I'd place my bet on someone who inherits good genes and who doesn't ruin good joints and healthy hearts by overuse. My Mother entered her 94th year without ever running one block or doing one push up. But she was thin and active. I doubt that exercise would have added one week to her longevity. And I also don't believe lions would live any longer if they wore Nike running shoes.

I believe one reason I got to 90+ was by walking to work in snow or rain every day and being involved in a sport such as tennis, that I enjoyed for years. But I never enjoyed repetitive exercise. I admit I now lift weights several times a day at my desk while writing. But I don't like it. I do it because my trap shooting shotgun gun weighs 7.5 pounds and I've learned I need strong arms to lift it and shoot 100 rounds!

Pitfalls of Exercise

Who Says 10,000 Steps a Day?

Walking has always been high priority for me. But how many steps do most people take daily, and how many are needed for good health? I had no idea how many I take and thought it would be interesting and prudent to find out. And who is right about exercise, Mark Twain or the Earl of Derby?

The first step was to purchase a pedometer. It's a small battery operated device (the cost about $35.00) that fits on the hip and counts your steps. Mine has more gizmos than I need. But the main button counts steps and another the calories burned up.

For years my normal day involved a 25 minute walk to my office and the same route home in late afternoon. During the day I never ran a marathon in the office but I also never slept on the couch. So I could hardly wait to open the pedometer to see how I had fared. The final tab: 9,100 steps. Studies show that most people take from 3,000 to 5,000 steps daily. This is a bit short of the 10,000 steps we're supposed to take. Or are we?

I discovered it was the Japanese who came up with this figure, and there's nothing magic about it. Rather, the number was used as a smart marketing device in a campaign to sell pedometers. But even though it was a smart sales move, medical authorities have agreed the proposed Japanese figure of 10,000 steps is a healthy number to aim for. But it does mean walking a hefty five miles.

So how many calories does 10,000 steps burn up? Let's say you've enjoyed a lunch of a double burger, fries and a sugar-loaded 10 ounce soft drink. This packs a caloric wallop of about 1,700 calories.

That's when the pedometer sends bad news. You will be surprised at the small number of calories you've burned up after a brisk walk. For instance, a 150 pound person, after 10,000 steps, loses only 500 calories.

So how do we burn up the remaining calories? Our Basal Metabolic Rate eats up 60 percent of our daily energy to keep all our organs functioning. Another 10 percent is required to absorb, digest and store food.

But why even buy a pedometer when we know that walking is good for you? Researchers I talked to stressed that counting steps with a pedometer is a great motivator and has more psychological impact than counting miles. But although stepping it up helps to lose weight, it will never win the battle of the bulge without the help of sound nutrition.

I found that knowing I walk 9,100 steps in an average day pushed me to see how much I could "step up" my own activity. It's easy to do. You can go for a walk at lunch. Or get off the bus a few blocks from home. The end result will be improved health.

Dr. Paul Dudley White, Harvard's renowned cardiologist who treated President Dwight Eisenhower's coronary attack, was a firm believer in "stepping-it-up." He taught that exercise had major physical and emotional advantages and that "If you want to know how flabby your brain is, feel your leg muscles!"

Some companies and organizations are encouraging members to make 10,000 steps their goal. But how many steps are needed depends on your age and health. And remember that walking is free, simple and convenient. Moreover, there's no need to break the record of the one-minute mile or purchase expensive exercise machines.

There's never been a better time to stress the health benefits of walking. It's been proven to help fight obesity, heart disease, diabetes, arthritis, osteoporosis, and strengthens muscles.

But exercise has always been a tough sell. Mark Twain claimed he'd been at the funerals of many friends who believed in exercise more than he did. But I believe the Earl of Derby was right when he remarked, "Those who do not find time for exercise will have to find time for illness." Amen to that.

Pitfalls of Infection

Pleasures and Dangers of Hot Tub Baths

So you've just checked into a hotel, gone to the health club in dire need of relaxation? So now you're sitting in a hot tub and the world looks a lot better? Unfortunately, you should know there are pleasures and hazards to most things in life and hot tubs are no exception. One of the hazards is "Hot Tub Lung Infection." If you're a woman, think again before you make the plunge. Remember you're often taking a bath with others. This is why it has never been high priority for me.

Perhaps as you were reaching to turn on the jets you saw this message out of the corner of your eye, "Persons suffering from heart disease, high blood pressure, diabetes, or other health problems should not enter the spa without prior medical consultation and permission from your doctor." There may also be warnings not to consume alcohol, use temperatures over 104 degrees, and if pregnant, consult a physician first.

In today's litigation-riddled society, this caution helps to ward off lawsuits. After all, when McDonalds can be sued if you spill a cup of hot coffee while driving and burn yourself, there's small wonder for such messages. But what is lurking in a hot tub?

It's hard to find a better place for bacteria and fungus infection to survive than a hot, wet area. This is why skin infection such as folliculitis can occur. But one bacterium, Mycobacterium avium, has a special liking for this location. This is particularly true if tubs are not cleaned as recommended by health authorities. And chlorine loses some of its effectiveness at temperatures above 84 degrees F.

But how can a germ in the water get into your lungs? Bubbles form in the contaminated water from the force of hot tub jets. These bubbles burst when they rise to the surface dispersing the bacteria into the air.

Mycobacterium avium is related to the class of bacteria that causes tuberculosis, but luckily it's not contagious. It can, however, cause fever or chills, a wet cough, tightness of the chest, fatigue and shortness of breath.

Diagnosis of Hot Tub Lung Infection is made by chest X-rays of the lungs. Testing water in the tub will also detect this bacterium. The usual treatment consists of corticosteroids and antibiotics to combat the inflammation and infection. Fortunately, this is not a common infection.

What is the risk of heart attack while using a hot tub? Some authorities are concerned that hot water could cause extra stress on the heart by increasing the heart rate.

Dr. Thomas Allison, a cardiologist at the Mayo Clinic, says that the chance of this happening is "pretty rare." But he advises that a stay in the tub should not last more than 15 minutes.

Other cardiologists suggest that patients who are taking beta-blockers and ACE inhibitors which lower blood pressure should use hot tubs cautiously. They should be aware of the risk of fainting after a long hot soak.

Sitting in a hot tub also causes blood vessels to dilate as the body adjusts to increased heat. This would normally cause a decrease in blood pressure as widened vessels mean less pressure is needed to push blood through the body. But the force of water against the body prevents this from happening. Stepping out of the tub removes this counterforce. In addition, gravity allows blood to drop towards the feet and as the brain loses blood, fainting may occur.

Deaths have been reported due to heat stroke from prolonged hot tub soaks. Being immersed for a long time prevents the body from sweating to remove excess heat.

It's debatable if hot tubs could cause damage to a developing fetus. But there's been enough concern expressed that in all probability pregnant women should forgo this pleasure. It's also easy for water to enter the vagina resulting in troublesome itchy fungus infection.

Urinary tract infections (UTIs) have been linked to hot tubs for one good reason. The anal area and bowel are home to E. Coli bacteria, the organism that causes most UTIs. Since the rectum is close to the vagina and urinary tract, contamination of urinary opening is always a possibility.

For the majority of people a few minutes in a hot tub is safe and beneficial. And for those suffering from arthritis, it helps to ease stiff joints and tight muscles by increasing blood flow and loosening connective tissue. But enjoy without alcohol. Imbibing makes you more likely to ignore warnings, become overheated and increases the risk of slipping.

Pitfalls of Infection

In Europe, Nobody Chides "We Know Where You're Going"

Have you ever heard of UTI Drops (urinary tract infection drops?). I doubt it as these natural herbal drops have just been imported from Europe to treat troublesome acute and chronic E Coli urinary tract infection. UTI Drops have been used successfully in Europe for over 20 years and have now been approved by Health Canada. So why are these natural herbs so effective in combating E. Coli, the bacteria that's responsible for most cases of bladder infection (cystitis)?

Every year 30 to 50 million North Americans, mostly women, the elderly, and those with compromised immune systems, suffer from cystitis. Few ever forget the first attack of severe pain on urination, fever and the constant rushing to the bathroom or the constant worry about the next attack. Then, the sheer terror if blood appears in the urine.

Urinary infections can be due to a variety of causes. Some are the result of a fallen bladder due to difficult childbirth which leaves stagnant urine in the bladder. Others result from the ring around the bathtub. Or the shortness of the urethra (the tube that carries urine from the bladder to the outside) in women makes it easier for E Coli to enter the bladder. And sexual intercourse is another factor.

So how do you prevent friends from chiding, "We know where

you're going." A good prevention is to take showers rather than baths and to urinate following sex.

Don't ignore your Mother's advice. For years, doctors "pooh-poohed" her theory that cranberry juice prevented UTI. But Harvard researchers proved she was right. They discovered that E. Coli bacteria have hair-like projections that enable them to stick to the bladder wall allowing them to multiply. Cranberry juice has an anti-sticking factor that prevents this so E. Coli are flushed out during urination.

Dr. Michael Weisspapir, Medical Director of Eastgate Pharmaceutical, says UTI Drops were created by Dr. Enes Hasanagic, a Yugoslavian herbal expert. He adds that the product is more effective than cranberry juice because, in addition to the anti-sticking factor, it has antibacterial and antiseptic properties, and also forms a protective layer on the walls of the urinary tract to prevent further bacterial growth.

Weisspapir explains that many remedies have low bioavailability. This means they do not absorb well and a high dose must be used to make them effective. But when the higher dose is required, there's greater risk of side-effects.

Eastgate technology overcomes this problem by a process called "self-emulsifying composition" and "Nano technology." This technique increases solubility and produces a final extract 200 to 1,000 times smaller than the human red blood cell. This makes UTI Drops highly absorbable so patients receive a low but still effective dose.

UTI drops are also preferable to antibiotics which often kill good bacteria and cause troublesome side-effects such as irritating yeast infections or allergic reactions. Today antibiotics have been so overused to treat recurrent urinary infections that they have become less effective.

The recommended dose of UTI Drops is 20 drops diluted in

a quarter of a glass of water, mixed well and drunk three times a day. It does not contain dairy products, wheat, gluten, yeast, corn, sugar or artificial colouring or flavouring. It should not be used if you are pregnant or have severe kidney disease. For males, twice the dose is usually required.

There's an old saying that, "if you don't go when you gotta go, by the time you go, you've already gone!" UTI Drops should end this problem and fewer people will hear the chiding words, "We know where you're going!"

UTI Drops will also ease the frustration of doctors who have patients returning for recurring urinary infections.

The longer I practiced medicine the more I realized that natural remedies were safer than man-made prescription drugs. Every year 100,000 North Americans die from prescription medication. Another 700,000 are admitted to emergency departments for drug complications.

Today, it makes sense that this natural herbal remedy, tested by time should be tried before drugs are prescribed. UTI Drops fills this need. Moreover, this remedy fulfills two important rules in medicine. First, do no harm. Second, keep it simple.

Pitfalls of Government Bureaucracy

Health Canada and CBC Television Distort Medical Facts

Do you remember the movie "Network?" Howard Beale (played by Peter Finch) is the evening news anchor on national TV and he's depressed about corruption, crime, unemployment and other societal ills. So angry, he decides to speak his mind during the evening broadcast, to everyone's surprise. Finally, after raving about injustices he shouts, "I'm mad as hell and I'm not gong to take it anymore" repeatedly. Then Beale tells listeners to go to their windows and shout, "I'm mad as hell and I'm not going to take it anymore."

This week, like Beale, I'm also mad as hell. Why? Because I was commissioned to do a 30 second commercial on CBC about a product I support called Medi-C Plus. Research has shown that this combination of high doses of vitamin C and lysine can save countless lives from heart attack, stroke and other cardiovascular complications. But according to rules established by the Canadian Ministry of Health, I could only say this product was helpful for bones, teeth and gums. This part is correct, but it belies the truth. Besides, no one could provide a logical reason for the prohibition. The product's main purpose is to prevent the nation's number one killer – heart attack. So why wouldn't this censure make me mad as hell!

This commercial was not promoting snake oil. It was reporting a life-saving product based on the research of Dr. Linus Pauling, two-time Nobel Prize winner. His research showed that vitamin C is essential to produce collagen, a glue that holds coronary cells together. And without large amounts of vitamin C and lysine, microscopic cracks occur in coronary arteries, the prelude to heart attack.

Dr. Sydney Bush, an England researcher, has since proven that this combination not only prevents atherosclerosis (hardening of arteries), but also reverses it. Moreover, he has photos taken over a 16-year period as proof. Photos are worth more than a thousand questionable statistical studies. Bush deserves the Nobel Prize for this research.

The censors at Health Canada should have done some homework before making their ludicrous decision. They don't need to be doctors to see the dramatic affect that vitamin C has on Bush's before-and-after photo. See my web site www.docgiff to see the photo.

This decision makes me mad as hell for other reasons. Readers of my medical column are well aware of questionable medical ads on TV. Multinational organizations push cereals loaded with sugar that add to the frightening epidemic of obesity and Type 2 diabetes. Cholesterol lowering drugs (CLDs) that are supposed to be the be-all-and-end-all of heart attack prevention, yet are associated with unintended and bothersome consequences. Yet I'm prevented from reporting the truth about a natural remedy that is effective, less expensive than a CLD, and has never killed anyone. Health Canada's regulation is a blatant distortion of scientific facts and a perfect example of thoughtless, bone-headed inconsistency.

This is a situation where it would be helpful if Canadian doctors were supportive, particularly cardiologists. But it hasn't happened. It is ironic that in spite of research studies, my columns, radio and TV interviews, and lectures across Canada, the medical establishment remains silent. Normally, in the past, when I have tackled controversial subjects, critical comments are triggered immediately. In this case, it appears there is no ammunition to fire.

Recently I watched the movie Network a second time. Again it made a good point. More of us should get mad as hell for asinine bureaucracy.

Needless to say I intend to protest this arbitrary and illogical ruling by Health Canada. I'm sure mine will be a lone voice. But in the end the general public often sees the falsehood of censorship.

Unfortunately, millions have died in the past because of the closed minds of doctors. Now, in 2015, how long will it take for Health authorities and doctors to accept that high doses of vitamin C and lysine can not only prevent, but also reverse, hardening of arteries, and end coronary attack from being the number one killer?

Pitfalls of Government Bureaucracy

My Number is 18924

Why am I mad as hell? I've joined "Dignitas," the Swiss organization that allows freedom of choice in death. Now I'm Registered Member 18924. I hope I don't get a chance to use my membership soon, or ever. But if I develop a debilitating illness, Dignitas' services will be available to me. Many share my view. But we all want to cry out "We're mad as hell and we're not going to take it anymore."

Let's first get mad as hell at gutless politicians, such as any Prime Minister who claims our Charter of Rights and Freedoms protects us all from injustice, yet denies freedom from the agony of terminal cancer pain, Lou Gehrig's Disease and other degenerative diseases. Some justice!

Then let's get mad as hell at those who constantly oppose assisted death for anyone, for selfish reasons. The ones who claim they have a superior moral code that the rest of us are lacking. Or insist that assisted death leads to the slippery slope theory of the elderly and crippled being arbitrarily removed from society for financial reasons.

These people should know this is a blatant lie. The truth is, and history has proven it, that people who are offered the choice of assisted death seldom use it. Rather, it's reassuring for them to know that this exit from life is available if they desperately need it.

I have no problem with those who, for religious, moral or ethical reasons, are opposed to assisted death for themselves. They have my blessing to suffer the agonies of painful death as long as they like. But they have no inborn right to say the rest of us are morally corrupt when deciding this is senseless torture.

So why am I complaining? There should be an even playing field. The choice to end one's life when terminal agony warrants it should be available to any who can't afford to purchase a one-way plane ticket to Switzerland, or do not wish to die in another country. This is where our Charter of Rights and Freedoms fails miserably.

As I write this book the Supreme Court is once again debating whether to allow assisted death in Canada. It's been said that war is too vital to be left in the hands of generals. History shows that the decision of assisted death is too important to be left in the hands of lawyers. Surveys prove the majority of Canadians want the option of assisted suicide. Hopefully, the learned judges will hear this message and legalize assisted death so there will be no need to purchase a one way ticket to Zurich.

What I and others ask for is freedom of choice in death. I have no desire to have physicians prolong my life when I decide otherwise. Today, many doctors lack commonsense. They are out of touch with reality when ordering procedures and tests in the final days of life that merely prolong agony. As Alexander the Great lamented centuries ago, "I die with the help of too many physicians."

Pitfall the Final One

It's Been a Great Ride

At 90+ I calculate that during my career as a medical journalist I've written over 2,500,000 words. It's been a privilege to be able to write them. After all, how many people can sit at a computer, express an opinion, and have over six million people read it, 52 weeks a year for 38 years? I thank my many editors, particularly those who did not fire me.

I doubt that history will memorialize what I have said over the years. But to the best of my ability, my words have been honest and I hope they have helped patients and readers.

I'm often asked whether I would now change my views. This question refers to the many controversial medical issues I've tackled. At times they made life difficult for me and my family. But in retrospect, avoidance would have been hard to do. The safe route would have been hypocritical. Some issues were too important to pass over and I have never been a fence-sitter. So I agree with the Periclean dictum, "In Athens we think that silent men are useless."

I would like to thank all of my colleagues at Preferred Nutrition for their friendship, support and hard work over the last two years.

Deane Parkes, President of Preferred Nutrition has been especially supportive and a great companion. I admire his creative insight and passion. And I am very appreciative of his effort and that of his team in the marketing of Medi-C Plus.

I wish to express a huge thanks to my wife, Susan, for her support and editorial help for 57 years. And for my children and grandchildren I hope this planet will be kind to them. Unfortunately, I believe it is on a collision course with nature and eventually Mother Nature may win.

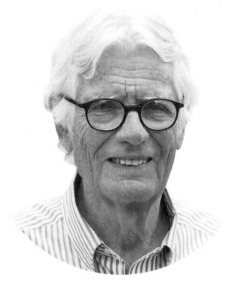

Sign up for my FREE health tips at www.docgiff.com